Mehdi Karoui
Ghassene Amri

Bipolar Disorder With Rapid Cycles

Mehdi Karoui

Ghassene Amri

Bipolar Disorder With Rapid Cycles

Clinical and therapeutic features

ScienciaScripts

Imprint

Any brand names and product names mentioned in this book are subject to trademark, brand or patent protection and are trademarks or registered trademarks of their respective holders. The use of brand names, product names, common names, trade names, product descriptions etc. even without a particular marking in this work is in no way to be construed to mean that such names may be regarded as unrestricted in respect of trademark and brand protection legislation and could thus be used by anyone.

Cover image: www.ingimage.com

This book is a translation from the original published under ISBN 978-620-3-44053-9.

Publisher:
Sciencia Scripts
is a trademark of
Dodo Books Indian Ocean Ltd. and OmniScriptum S.R.L publishing group

120 High Road, East Finchley, London, N2 9ED, United Kingdom
Str. Armeneasca 28/1, office 1, Chisinau MD-2012, Republic of Moldova, Europe
Printed at: see last page
ISBN: 978-620-6-12508-2

Copyright © Mehdi Karoui, Ghassene Amri
Copyright © 2023 Dodo Books Indian Ocean Ltd. and OmniScriptum S.R.L publishing group

Contents

I. INTRODUCTION

Bipolar disorder (BD) is a chronic, frequent and particularly severe psychiatric condition with significant morbidity and mortality [1]. It is one of the main causes of disability worldwide, especially in young people. Patients with TB suffer substantial impairment of function for most of their lives, particularly as a result of depression [2].

Although described as far back as antiquity, the notion of bipolar disorder emerged during the 19eme century. It was called "circular madness" by Falret in 1851, "double-form madness" by Baillarger in 1854 and "manic-depressive madness" by Kraepelin in 1899. The term "bipolar psychosis" appeared later with Kleist in 1953 [3,4].

It was not until 1980, with the DSM-III, that manic-depressive psychosis was officially separated into two distinct entities: unipolar and bipolar. The term manic-depressive psychosis was then replaced by bipolar disorder [5].

The prevalence of TB is estimated at between 1 and 2.5% of the population [6]. In parallel with the increase in its frequency, we have seen a broadening of its spectrum. It thus goes far beyond the standard form of manic-depressive psychosis, incorporating dimensions such as polarity and recurrence.

This is how rapid cycles come into being, as one of the evolutionary modes of TB. This entity is still poorly defined. It may occur at the onset of the disorder or may become chronic [7].

The term "rapid cycling" was first introduced in 1974 by Dunner and Fieve when they worked with patients who showed a poor response to lithium salts and in whom they recorded a high frequency of thymic recurrences [8].

Their definition was subsequently adopted by many clinicians and was introduced into the DSM-IV [9] as a clinical specification for bipolar disorder type 1 and type 2.

Rapid cycling (RC) is defined by the presence over the last twelve months of at least four thymic episodes meeting the criteria of a characteristic depressive, manic or hypomanic episode. The episodes are delimited by the occurrence of a complete or partial remission lasting at least two months or by the transition to an episode of opposite polarity [10].

The annual prevalence of rapid cycling in the clinical population is estimated at between 5 and 33.3%, while its lifetime prevalence is estimated at between 25.8 and 43% [11].

This clinical form has been associated by many authors with a predominance of type 2 bipolar disorder [12], depressive symptomatology [13] and female gender [14]. Its onset may be spontaneous or accelerated by the use of psychoactive substances [15]. An iatrogenic etiology has also been suggested to explain its appearance in some patients [16].

However, this evolutionary modality remains a poorly individualised entity in the literature. The profile of patients presenting with this clinical specification is poorly defined and the therapeutic options are poorly codified. Tunisian studies on this subject are rare.

This is the background to our study, which aims to :

-       To describe the sociodemographic and clinical characteristics of patients with rapid-cycling bipolar disorder.

-       To compare the sociodemographic, clinical and therapeutic characteristics of patients with bipolar disorder with rapid cycles with those of patients with bipolar disorder without rapid cycles.

II. PATIENTS AND METHODS

1. Type of study

This is a retrospective, descriptive and comparative study conducted among patients who were hospitalised at the Razi Hospital in La Manouba in the period from January 2015 to December 2017 and followed for bipolar disorder for at least two years.

2. Study location

The study was conducted in the "Avicenne" (A), "Pinel" (B) and "Ibn Jazzar" (G) psychiatric wards at the Razi Hospital in Manouba. These departments receive patients from the governorates of Beja, Seliana and Bizerte, as well as patients from the Greater Tunis delegations: Ariana, Ezzouhour, Hrairia, La Soukra, Le Bardo and Raoued for the psychiatry department (A), Carthage, Kalaat el-Andalous, La Marsa and Sidi Thabet for the psychiatry department (B) and Denden, Djebel Jelloud, El Ouardia, Kabaria, La Manouba and Oued Ellil for the psychiatry department (G).

3. Study population

Our work focused on a trained population of 97 patients followed for bipolar disorder diagnosed according to DSM-5 criteria. The patients were divided into two groups:

3.1. Rapid cycling bipolar disorder (RCBD) group: n= 37.

3.2. Group of patients with bipolar disorder without rapid cycling (TBNCR): n = 60.

3.3. Inclusion criteria

The rapid cycling group included individuals with bipolar disorder type 1 or type 2 who had at least four thymic episodes during a 12-month period that met the criteria for a typical depressive, manic or hypomanic episode as defined in the DSM-5.

3.4. Non-inclusion criteria

Patients with thymic episodes caused by a substance (e.g. cocaine, corticoids) or by another medical condition, patients with schizoaffective disorder and patients with cyclothymic disorder were not included in the study.

3.5. Exclusion criteria

Patients who had been treated for bipolar disorder for less than two years and those whose diagnosis of bipolar disorder had been revised were excluded from the study.

Patients whose files could not be used due to a lack of data to process were excluded.

4. Conduct of the survey

Sociodemographic data were collected from patients' medical records by consulting the list of hospital admissions from January 2015 to December 2017. We traced the clinical and developmental history of the disorder in the patients by establishing a chronology of thymic episodes and noting the clinical and therapeutic features of each episode from the date of onset of the disorder until the time of the study in December 2020 (Appendix 1).

5. Variables studied

5.1. Socio-demographic and biographical characteristics

We collected information on age, sex, place of residence, level of education, occupation and income. We also collected biographical data on family situation, such as parental consanguinity and parental divorce or death.

5.2. Family history

We looked for family psychiatric antecedents of mood disorders, psychosis, anxiety disorders, substance use disorders and suicide attempts, as well as family judicial antecedents.

5.3. Personal history and habits

Personal habits of consumption of psychoactive substances, in particular alcohol, cannabis, psychotropic drugs, injectable substances, volatile solvents and amphetamines, were investigated, as well as any history of childhood sexual abuse or maltreatment and the presence of self-mutilation or tattoos. The existence of judicial antecedents was also collected. We also looked for somatic antecedents.

5.4. Clinical parameters

The general clinical data collected concerned the main psychiatric diagnosis (type 1 or type 2 bipolar disorder). For each patient we traced the history of the thymic illness by collecting the age of onset of the index episode and its polarity, the total number of thymic episodes, manic, depressive and hypomanic episodes, the predominant polarity (defined by the threshold of two thirds or more of the thymic episodes on a single pole on a lifetime count of episodes [17]), the number of hospitalisations and the mean length of hospitalisation.

For each thymic episode, we recorded the clinical characteristics as specified in the DSM-5, i.e. the presence of psychotic features, mixed features, melancholic features, atypical features, catatonia, peripartum onset and seasonality.

5.5. Therapeutic parameters

We collected the molecules prescribed in each patient's file since their first thymic episode and classified them as tricyclic antidepressants, serotonin reuptake inhibitors, serotonin and noradrenaline reuptake inhibitors, lithium salts, anticonvulsants, classic antipsychotics, atypical antipsychotics, clozapine, benzodiazepines, antihistamine-type hypnotics or zolpidem. We also noted any use of electro-convulsive therapy or transcranial magnetic stimulation.

6. Data analysis

The data were entered and analysed using IBM SPSS Statistics 22 software.

6.1. Descriptive study

For qualitative variables, we calculated absolute frequencies and relative frequencies (percentages). For each quantitative variable, we calculated the mean, median and standard deviation and determined the extreme values.

6.2. Analytical study

Comparisons of two means on independent series were carried out using Student's *t-test* for independent series.

Comparisons of percentages on independent series were made using Pearson's *chi-square* test. If this test was invalid, the comparison of two percentages was carried out using Fisher's two-tailed exact test.

In all statistical tests, the significance level was set at 0.05.

7. Bibliographic research

The identification of the variables to be studied and the discussion of our results were based on a search for similar studies in scientific literature or published in specialist scientific journals, as well as on reports from international bodies interested in this subject.

Our bibliographic search was based on the following key words: "mood disorder", "bipolar disorder", "manic episodes", "bipolar depression", "rapid cycles", "epidemiology", "evolution", "prognosis" and "complications".

We searched the following scientific databases: Embase (Elsevier), Med-line (PubMed), Clinicalkey, Science direct, Google scholar, Scopus, Em-consulte and Springer.

8. Ethical considerations and conflicts of interest

The anonymity of the patients has been respected for each file collected. We declare that we have no conflict of interest in relation to this work.

III. RESULTS

1. Descriptive study

The group of patients with rapid cycling bipolar disorder (RCBD) numbered n=37 and represented 38.14% of the total study population (n=97).

1.1. Socio-demographic data

1.1.1. Age

The mean age of the patients was 41.08 years, with a standard deviation of 10.887 years and extremes of 22 and 79 years.

1.1.2. The genre

The TBCR group comprised 25 male and 12 female patients. The sex ratio was 2.08 (Figure 1).

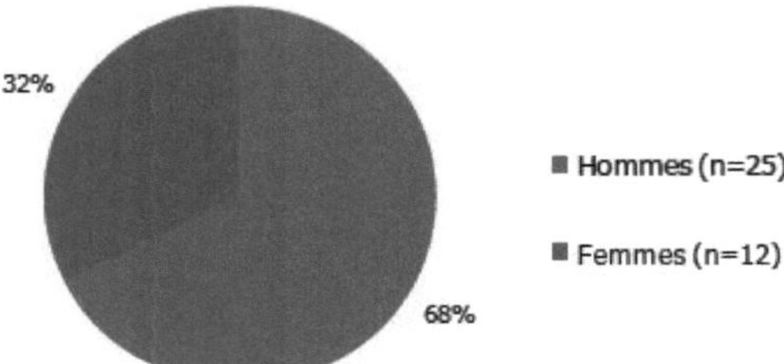

Figure 1. Gender distribution of TBCR patients

1.1.3. Place of residence

Patients living in urban areas represented 75.7% of the population studied (n=28). Those living in Greater Tunis accounted for more than half the patients (n=19) (Figure 2).

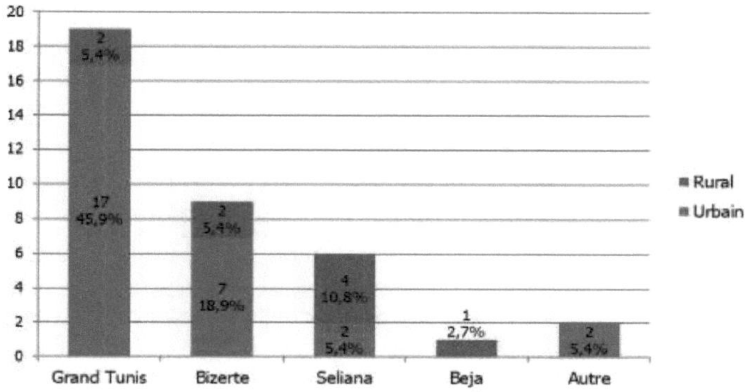

Figure 2. Lieu de résidence des patients TBCR

1.1.4. Parents' status

Parental consanguinity was found in 27% of patients (n=10) and parental divorce in 10.8% (n=4). The death of at least one parent was noted in 40% of TBCR patients (n=15).

1.1.5. Level of education and vocational training

In the TBCR patient population, 12 patients had a primary level of education, representing 32.4% of the sample. Those with secondary education were 19 and represented 51.4%. Six patients or 16.2% of the sample had higher education. Six patients (16.2%) had vocational training (Figure 3).

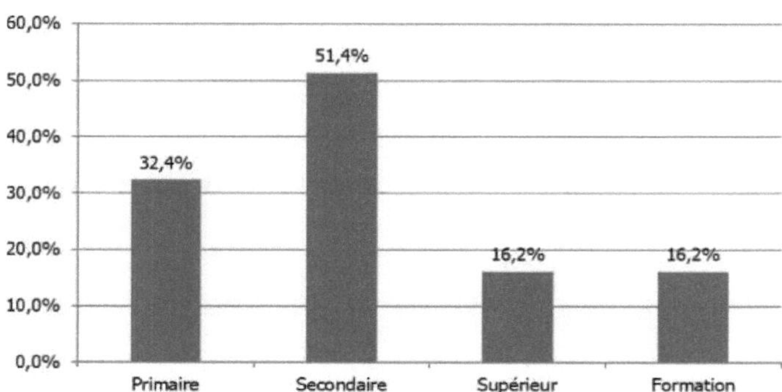

Profess io nal

Figure 3: Level of education among TBCR patients

1.1.6. Professional activity

In the population studied, 97.3% of patients had no professional activity (Figure 4).

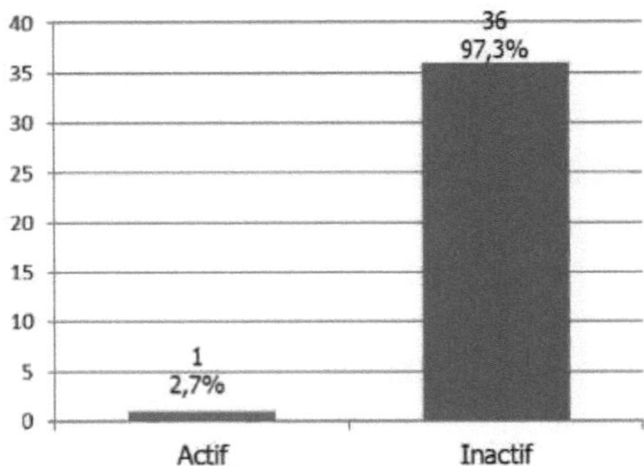

Figure 4: Occupational status of TBCR patients

1.1.7. Socio-economic level

The income level was average for 73% of patients (n=27). Patients with a low income represented 18.9% of the sample (n=7) and those with a high income (n=3) represented 8.1%.

1.1.8. Marital status

In the population studied, 48.6% of patients were single (n=18), 40.5% were married (n=15) and 10.8% were divorced (n=4).

The majority of patients, 94.6% (n=35), lived with a close relative. Only one patient was living with distant relatives and only one was in a residential institution.

1.2. Family background

A family history of a mood disorder was found in 43.2% of TBCR patients (n=16) and a family history of a psychotic disorder in 18.9% (n=7). Anxiety disorders were present in the family histories of 8.1% of patients (n=3) and substance use disorder in those of 10.8% (n=4). Three patients (8.1%) had a family history of suicide attempts (Figure 5). Two patients (5.4%) had a family history of incarceration.

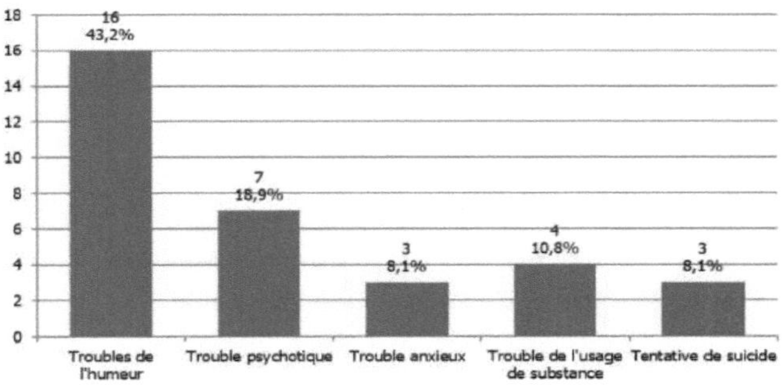

Figure 5. Psychiatric family antecedents of TBCR patients

1.3. Personal history

1.3.1. Personal history of somatic illness

Cardiovascular and metabolic antecedents were noted in 27% of patients in the study population (n=10): arterial hypertension in two patients, diabetes in two patients, dyslipidemia in one patient, obesity in six patients and coronary artery disease in one patient.

Infectious diseases were found, notably tuberculosis in two patients and viral hepatitis in one.

Vitiligo was reported in one patient and psoriasis in two others.

1.3.2. Personal history of psychoactive substance use

Regular alcohol consumption was found in 59.5% of patients (n=22). Cannabis was found in 37.8% (n=14).

Ten TBCR patients (27%) had personal habits of psychotropic drug use, and two patients (5.4%) used volatile solvents. Only one patient (2.7%) had a personal history of amphetamine use. None of the TBCR patients had a history of injectable substance use (Figure 6).

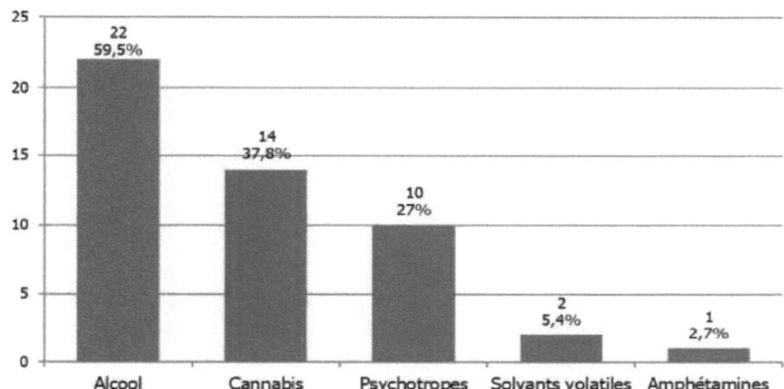

Figure 6. Use of psychoactive substances by patients with CRBT

1.3.3. Personal history of sexual abuse and mistreatment

A personal history of sexual abuse was reported in 8.1% of TBCR patients (n=3) and maltreatment in 21.6% (n=8).

1.3.4. Personal history of tattoos or self-mutilation

Tattoos and self-mutilation were present in 10 patients, i.e. 27% of the population studied.

1.3.5. Personal legal history

A history of incarceration or arrest was noted in 29.7% of the population studied (n=11).

1.4. Clinical data

1.4.1. Main diagnosis of bipolar disorder

Bipolar disorder type 1 was present in 94.6% of patients (n=35). Two patients were diagnosed with bipolar disorder type 2.

1.4.2. Age of onset of disorder

The mean age of onset was 23.73 years, with a standard deviation of 5.91 and extremes of 13 and 42 years.

1.4.3. Polarity of the index episode

In 56.8% of patients, the index episode was of the depressive type (n=21). A manic or hypomanic index episode was noted in 43.2% of patients (n=16).

1.4.4. Number of episodes

TBCR patients had a mean of 13.95 thymic episodes of all polarities, with a standard deviation of

7.746.

The mean number of manic episodes was 9.35 with a standard deviation of 8.11. The mean number of depressive episodes was 4.22 with a standard deviation of 3.743, and the mean number of hypomanic episodes was 0.38 with a standard deviation of 0.639.

Manic polarities were dominant in 56.76% of patients (n=21) and depressive polarities in 27.03% (n=10) (Figure 7).

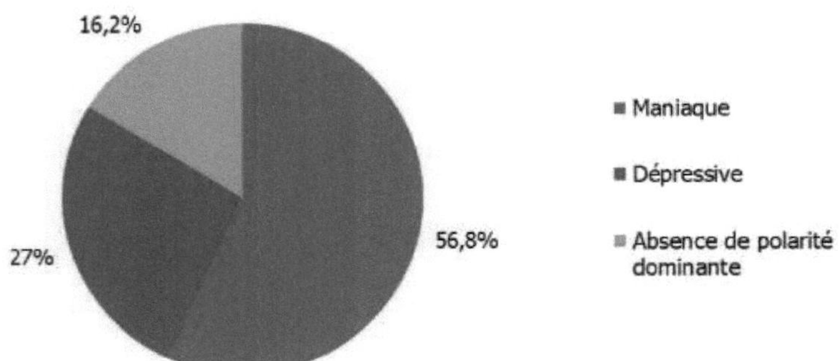

Figure 7. Dominant potarite in TBCR patients

1.4.5. Hospital admissions

The mean number of hospital admissions was 10.51 with a standard deviation of 6.11. The mean length of hospital stay was 17.95 days, with a standard deviation of 7.60. TBCR patients therefore spent an average of 195.95 days in hospital, with a standard deviation of 146.66.

1.4.6. Clinical characteristics of thymic episodes

TBCR patients presented an average of 9.24 thymic episodes with psychotic features, 1.57 thymic episodes with mixed features, 1.27 thymic episodes with anxiety distress, 0.95 thymic episodes with melancholic features, 1.35 thymic episodes with atypical features and 0.08 thymic episodes with catatonia.

The seasonal nature of the disorders was found in 16.2% of patients (n=6).

Five TBCR patients (41.6%) had a thymic episode with onset during the peripartum period. The mean number of these episodes was 0.5 (Table I).

Table I Characteristics of thymic episodes in TBCR *patients*

	Mean (standard deviation) [Min - Max]	
Thymic episode with :		
Psychotic features	9,24 (7,686)	[0 - 32]
Mixed characteristics	1,57 (2,007)	[0 - 9]
Anxiety distress	1,27 (1,521)	[0 - 5]
Melancholic characteristics	0,95 (1,731)	[0 - 6]
Atypical features	1,35 (2,831)	[0 - 14]
Catatonia	0,08 (0,277)	[0 - 1]
Early peri-partum	0,50 (0,674)	[0 - 2]

1.4.7. Psychiatric comorbidities

Psychiatric comorbidity was present in more than half of the population studied (n=21). Alcohol and cannabis use disorders were present in 10.81% and 21.62% of patients respectively (n=4 and n=8). A personality disorder was present in 21.62% of patients (n=8). An anxiety disorder was present in one patient (Figure 8).

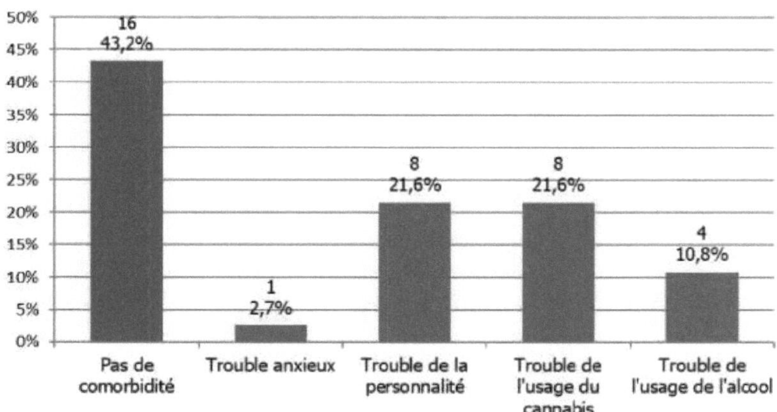

Figure 8. Psychiatric comorbidities in CRBT patients

1.4.8. Suicide attempts

Suicide attempts were reported in 19 patients, i.e. 51.4% of the population. The mean number of suicide attempts per patient was 2.16, with a standard deviation of 2.089 and extremes between 1 and 10.

In the TBCR group, the mean number of suicide attempts was 1.11, with a standard deviation of 1.838 and extremes between 0 and 10.

1.5. Therapeutic data

1.5.1. Treatment with antidepressants

Treatment with tricyclic antidepressants was noted in 13.5% of patients (n=5). Serotonin reuptake inhibitors were used in 37.8% of patients (n=14) and serotonin and noradrenaline reuptake inhibitors in 8.1% of patients (n=3).

1.5.2. Treatment with anticonvulsants

All TBCR patients (n=37) received at least one anticonvulsant. Sodium valproate was used in 81.1% of patients (n=30), carbamazepine in 81.1% of patients (n=30) and lamotrigine in

24.3% of patients (n=9).

1.5.3. Lithium treatment

Lithium was used in 18.9% of patients (n=7).

1.5.4. Treatment with neuroleptics

Classic neuroleptics were used by 83.8% of patients (n=31) and atypical neuroleptics by 83.8% (n=31).

1.5.5. Treatment with clozapine

Only one patient was put on clozapine.

1.5.6. Treatment with benzodiazepines

Benzodiazepines were used in 83.8% of patients (n=31).

1.5.7. Treatment with hypnotics

Antihistamines or zolpidem were used in 56.8% of patients (n=21).

1.5.8. Treatment with electroconvulsive therapy

Only one patient in our series was treated with electroconvulsive therapy (ECT).

1.5.9. Transcranial magnetic stimulation treatment

Repetitive transcranial magnetic stimulation (RTMS) was used in three patients, representing 8.1% of the population studied.

2. Comparative study
2.1. Socio-demographic data

2.1.1. Age

There was no statistically significant difference between the mean ages of the TBCR (41.08) and TBNCR (42.67, p=0.495) patient groups.

2.1.2. The genre

The sex ratio in the TBCR group was 2.08 and in the TBNCR group 1.72. The gender distribution was not significantly different between the two groups of patients. (p=0,671)

2.1.3. Place of residence

The TBNCR group included 81.7% of individuals living in urban areas (n=49) and 18.3% of individuals living in rural areas (n=11). There was no statistically significant difference with the TBCR group (p=0.479).

2.1.4. Parents' status

We found no statistically significant differences between the TBCR and TBNCR groups with regard to consanguinity, parental death or divorce.

2.1.5. Level of education and vocational training

In the TBNCR group, patients with primary education represented 40% of the study population (n=24). Those with secondary and university education represented 46.7% and 13.3% respectively (n=28 and n=8). There was no statistically significant difference with the group of TBCR patients (p=0.745).

Nor did we find any statistically significant difference between the two groups in terms of vocational training (p=0.233).

2.1.6. Professional activity

The rate of patients with no work activity was significantly higher (**p=0.015**) in the TBCR group than in the TBNCR group (Figure 9).

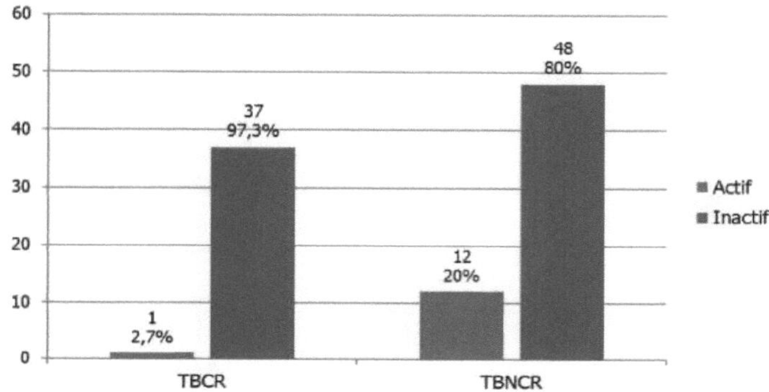

Figure 9. Com pa reason for 'professional activity' in TBCR and TBNCR patients

2.1.7. Income level

Patients with low income in the TBNCR group represented 30% of the sample (n=18). The difference with the TBCR group was not significant (p=0.226).

2.1.8. Marital status

In the TBNCR group, 51.7% of patients were single (n=31), 38.3% were married (n=23), 3.3% were divorced (n=2) and 6.7% were widowed (n=4).

We did not find any statistically significant difference between "married" and "unmarried" status, or between "divorced" and "non-divorced" status compared with the TBCR group.

2.2. Family background

2.2.1. Family psychiatric history

In the TBNCR group, we found a family history of bipolar disorder in 31.7% of patients (n=19), psychotic disorder in 28.3% (n=17), substance abuse in 3.3% (n=2) and attempted suicide in 8.3% (n=5). These differences were not statistically significant (Table II).

Table II Psychiatric family antecedents in TBCR and TBNCR patients

Variable	Patients with CR (*n* = 37)	Patients without CR (*n* = 60)	P
Family background n (%)			
Mood disorders	16 (43,2%)	19 (31,7%)	0,249
Psychotic disorders	7 (18,9%)	17 (28,3%)	0,297
Anxiety disorders	3 (8,1%)	0 (0%)	0,053
Substance use disorder	4 (10,8%)	2 (3,3%)	0,138
Suicide attempts	3 (8,1%)	5 (8,3%)	1,000

2.2.2. Judicial family history

A family history of incarceration was found in 8.3% of patients in the TBNCR group (n=5). There was no statistically significant difference with the TBCR group (p=0.705).

2.3. Personal history

2.3.1. Personal history of somatic illness

A comparison of the frequency of somatic pathologies in the two groups did not reveal any statistically significant differences.

2.3.2. Personal history of psychoactive substance use

Psychotropic drug use was significantly higher in the TBCR group (**p=0.046**). There were no statistically significant differences in the use of alcohol, cannabis, injection drugs, volatile solvents or amphetamines (Table III).

Tabieau III. Personal history of substance use in TBCR and TBNCR patients

Variable	Patients with CR (*n* = 37)	Patients without CR (*n* = 60)	*P*
Psychoactive substances			
Alcohol	22 (59,5%)	24 (40%)	0,062
Cannabis	14 (37,8%)	13 (21,7%)	0,084
Psychotropic drugs	10 (27%)	6 (10%)	**0,046**
Injectable substances	0 (0%)	2 (3,3%)	0,523
Volatile solvents	2 (5,4%)	0 (0%)	0,143
Amphetamines	1 (2,7%)	2 (3,3%)	1

2.3.3. Personal history of sexual abuse

A personal history of sexual abuse was found in 8.1% of TBCR patients (n=3) and in 1.7% of TBNCR patients (n=1). The difference was not statistically significant (p=0.154).

2.3.4. Personal history of abuse

Exposure to maltreatment was noted in 21.6% of TBCR patients (n=8) and in 13.3% of TBNCR patients (n=8). We found no statistically significant difference between the two groups (p=0.399).

2.3.5. Personal history of tattoos or self-mutilation

Personal history of tattooing or self-mutilation was significantly higher in the TBCR group (**p=0.028**).

2.3.6. Personal legal history

There was no statistically significant difference in the judicial antecedents of the two groups (p=0.129).

2.4. Clinical data

2.4.1. Main diagnosis of bipolar disorder

All patients in the TBNCR group had type 1 bipolar disorder. We found no statistically significant difference with the TBCR group.

2.4.2. Age of onset of disorder

There was no statistically significant difference between the mean age of onset of the disease in patients in the TBNCR group (26.02 years) and that in the TBCR group (23.73 years): p=0.107.

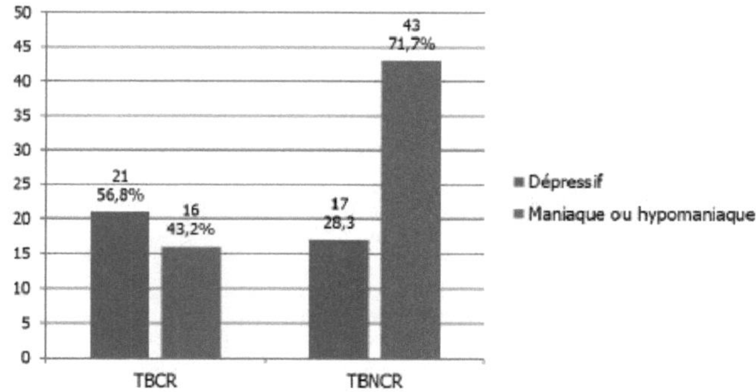

Figure 10. Polar map of the index episode in TBCR and TBNCR patients

2.4.3. Index episode

A depressive bias in the index episode was significantly more frequent in patients in the TBCR group: **p=0.005** (Figure 10).

2.4.4. Number of thymic episodes

Patients in the TBCR group had significantly more cumulative lifetime thymic episodes (**p=0.012**), more cumulative lifetime manic episodes (**p<0.001**) and more cumulative lifetime characteristic depressive episodes (**p<0.001**). There was no statistically significant difference in the mean number of hypomanic episodes (Figure 11).

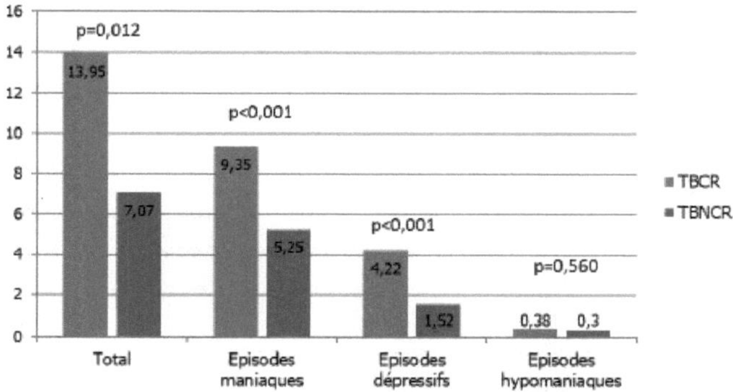

Figure 11. Average number of thymic episodes in TBCR and TBNCR patients

2.4.5. Dominant polarity

A dominant depressive polarity was found significantly more frequently in patients in the TBCR group (Figure 12): **p=0.017.**

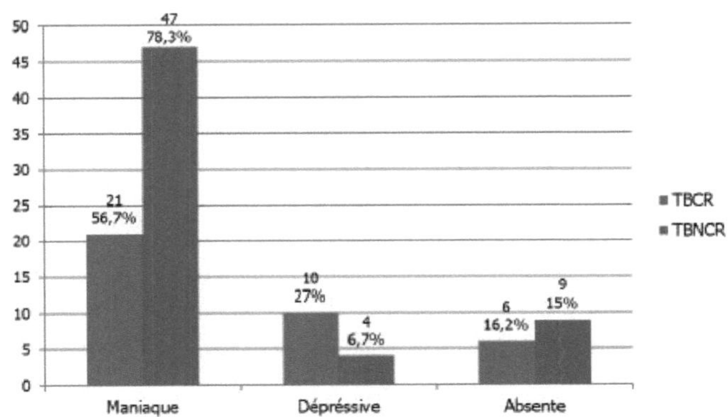

Figure 12. Dominant polarity in TBCR and TBNCR patients

2.4.6. Hospital admissions

The mean number of hospitalisations was statistically significantly higher in patients in the TBCR group (10.51 hospitalisations versus 4.72; **p<0.001**). We found no statistically significant difference between the mean lengths of stay in the two groups (p=0.165).

2.4.7. Clinical characteristics of thymic episodes

Patients in the TBCR group had statistically significantly more thymic episodes with melancholic features than patients in the TBNCR group (**p=0.022**). No statistically significant differences were found for psychotic features, mixed features, anxiety distress, atypical features, peripartum onset, catatonia and seasonality (Table VI).

Table IV. Comparison of the dynamic characteristics of thymic episodes

in TBCR and TBNCR patients

Variable	Patients with CR (n = 37)	Patients without CR (n = 60)	P
Clinical characteristics frequency (standard deviation)			
Psychotic features	62,08% (22,26)	62,88%(25,32)	0,875
Mixed characteristics	10,75% (11,23)	7,07% (11,95)	0,135
Anxiety distress	10,35% (14,53)	5,02% (10,00)	0,054
Melancholic characteristics	8,23% (15,16)	2,01% (6,34)	**0,022**
Atypical features	10,62% (18,89)	6,71% (12,72)	0,270
Catatonia	0,70% (2,53)	0% (0,00)	0,087
Early peri-partum	2,80% (4,01)	5,22% (9,00)	0,289

2.4.8. Psychiatric comorbidities

The presence of a psychiatric comorbidity was significantly more frequently associated with the presence of rapid cycles (**p=0.015**). No statistically significant difference was found when psychiatric disorders were compared individually (Table V).

Tabdeau V. Psychiatric comorbidities in TBCR and TBNCR patients

Variable	Patients with CR (n = 37)	Patients without CR (n = 60)	P

Psychiatric comorbidity n(%)	21 (56,8%)	19 (31,7%)	**0,015**
Anxiety disorders	1 (2,7%)	0 (0,0%)	0,381
Personality disorders	8 (21,62%)	5 (8,33%)	0,073
Cannabis use disorder	8 (21,62%)	5 (8,33%)	0,188
Alcohol use disorder	4 (10,81%)	7 (11,67%)	1,000

2.4.9. Suicide attempts

The occurrence of a suicide attempt was statistically significantly associated with the presence of rapid cycles: 51.4% of TBCR patients versus 13.3% of TBNCR patients (**p<0.001**) (Figure 13).

We found no statistically significant difference between the average number of suicide attempts.

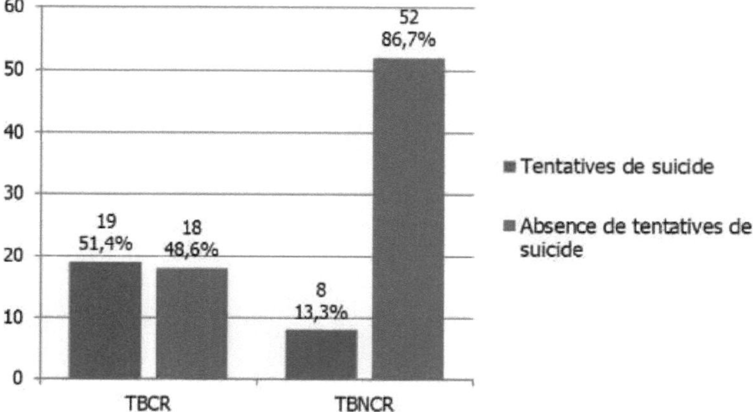

Figure 13. Prevalence of suicide attempts in TBCR and TBNCR patients

2.5. Therapeutic data

Prescription of serotonin reuptake inhibitors was significantly higher in patients in the TBCR group (**p=0.019**). We found no statistically significant differences for the other classes of antidepressants: serotonin and noradrenaline reuptake inhibitors and tricyclic antidepressants.

We found no statistically significant differences in the prescription of thymoregulators and antipsychotics.

The use of hypnotics such as antihistamines and zolpidem was significantly higher in the TBCR group (**p=0.009**) (Table VI).

Variable	Patients with CR ($n = 37$)	Patients without CR ($n = 60$)	P
Therapeutic data Tricyclic antidepressants	5 (13,5%)	4 (6,7%)	0,295
Serotonin reuptake inhibitors n (%)	14 (37,8%)	10 (16,7%)	**0,019**
Serotonin and noradrenaline reuptake inhibitors n (%)	3 (8,1%)	3 (5%)	0,671
Anticonvulsants n (%)	37 (100%)	58 (96,7%)	0,523
Lithium n (%)	7 (18,9%)	12 (20,0%)	0,896
Conventional neuroleptics n (%)	31 (83,8%)	56 (93,3%)	0,174
Atypical antipsychotics n (%)	31 (83,8%)	45 (75,0%)	0,308
Clozapine n (%)	1 (2,7%)	0 (0,0%)	0,381
Benzodiazepines n (%)	31 (83,8%)	47 (78,3%)	0,511
Hypnotics n (%)	31 (83,8%)	18 (30,0%)	**0,009**
ECT n (%)	1 (2,7%)	0 (0,0%)	0,381
RTMS n (%)	3 (8,1%)	0 (0,0%)	0,053

Table VI Treatment regimens for TBCR and TBNCR patients

IV. DISCUSSION

1. Main results

Our study first provided a sociodemographic, clinical and therapeutic description of the group of patients with bipolar disorder with rapid cycles, and then compared this group with a clinical population of patients with bipolar disorder who had never experienced rapid cycles.

The mean age at the time of the study was 41 years (+/- 10), with a sex ratio of 2.08. Three-quarters of the patients were from urban areas, with more than half living in Greater Tunis. Three quarters of the patients were from urban areas, with more than half living in the greater Tunis area.

One third of patients had primary education and half had secondary education. Patients with no professional activity represented 97% of the series.

Parental consanguinity was found in 27% of patients and parental divorce in 10%. Almost half the patients were single and 10% were divorced.

We noted family psychiatric antecedents of bipolar disorder, psychotic disorder, substance use disorders and suicide attempts in 43%, 18.9%, 10% and 8.1% of patients respectively.

Personal substance use habits were reported in 59.5% of patients for alcohol, 37.8% for cannabis and 27% for psychotropic drugs. More than a quarter of patients had self-mutilation or tattoos. One-fifth had been mistreated, and 8.1% were victims of abuse.

The majority of patients were being treated for type 1 bipolar disorder (94.6%). The index episode occurred at a mean age of 23.73 years (+/-5.9). This episode was depressive in 56.8% of cases.

The mean number of thymic episodes was 13.95, with a mean of 9.3 manic episodes, 4.22 depressive episodes and 0.38 hypomanic episodes. The mean number of hospital admissions was 10.5. The dominant polarity was manic in 56% of patients and depressive in 27%.

Psychotic features were noted in almost two-thirds of the thymic episodes. Atypical features, mixed features and anxiety distress were each present in 10% of episodes. Melancholic features were present in 8.1% of episodes.

More than half the patients had a psychiatric comorbidity. Alcohol use disorder was present in 10.81% of patients and cannabis use disorder in 21.62%. One-fifth of patients had an associated personality disorder.

More than half the patients had attempted suicide, with an average of 2.16 attempts per suicidal patient.

Therapeutically, tricyclic antidepressants were prescribed in 13.5% of patients and serotonin reuptake inhibitors in 37.8%. Both conventional and atypical antipsychotics were used in 83.8% of patients. All patients received anticonvulsants and 18.9% received lithium. Clozapine was used in only one patient. Electroconvulsive therapy and transcranial magnetic stimulation were used in one and three patients respectively.

Comparison of sociodemographic characteristics with the group of bipolar patients without rapid cycles showed no differences in mean age at the time of the study, or in gender, geographical origin or marital status. However, occupational inactivity was more frequent in patients with rapid cycles (p=0.015).

A higher proportion of patients with rapid cycling bipolar disorder had a history of alcohol, cannabis and psychotropic drug use. This difference was significant only for psychotropic drug use (p=0.046). These patients also had a greater frequency of self-mutilation and tattoos. The difference was statistically significant (p=0.028).

The average age of onset of their disease was 2.29 years earlier, but this difference was not statistically significant.

An index episode of depressive polarity (p=0.005) and a dominant depressive polarity (p=0.017) were more frequently found in the group of patients with rapid cycles. The total number of thymic episodes (p<0.001), manic episodes (p=0.006), characterised depressive episodes (p<0.001) and hospitalisations (p<0.001) was higher. Melancholic features were more often present (p=0.022).

Patients with rapid-cycling bipolar disorder had significantly more psychiatric comorbidities (p=0.015) and a higher frequency of suicide attempts (p<0.001).

From a therapeutic point of view, a significantly higher proportion of patients received treatment with serotonin reuptake inhibitor antidepressants (p=0.019) and antihistamine and zolpidem hypnotics (p=0.009) in the rapid cycling group.

2. Strengths and limitations

The interest of our study lies in having described a profile of patients presenting with a rarely individualised form of bipolar disorder. In fact, this work, which is both descriptive and comparative, has shed light on a population that is little studied in the literature. To our knowledge, it is the first study to focus on Tunisian patients with rapid-cycling bipolar disorder. It has made it possible to trace the long and heterogeneous course of the disorder and to determine its therapeutic and prognostic implications.

Our work must be interpreted with due regard for methodological limitations. These limitations are primarily related to the relatively small size of our sample, which constitutes an initial bias. A larger number of patients would have made our results more powerful and therefore more significant.

The retrospective nature of the study constitutes a second potential bias, due to lack of data or recall bias. In fact, certain parameters such as family antecedents, consumption habits or antecedents relating to early childhood could lack detail in certain observations. Data relating to the undesirable effects of the treatments received, such as neurological effects or effects on sexuality, were not systematically recorded.

Assessment of the quality of free time, socio-professional integration and level of income remained subjective. It depended on what the families said and on the assessment of the psychiatrist providing care.

In order to avoid some of these measurement biases, we excluded from the study imprecise records and records of patients whose follow-up had been interrupted.

Furthermore, our work includes a selection bias. Patients were recruited from the psychiatric departments of the Razi Hospital, which are subject to a sectorisation law. Thus, even if the population studied could come from five different governorates, our results are difficult to apply to all patients with bipolar disorder in Tunisia.

The fact that this study was carried out on inpatient wards at the Razi Hospital exposes another selection bias: the patients included in the study most often presented more severe symptoms of bipolar disorder. They were most often hospitalised for decompensations of type 1 bipolar disorder.

3. Sociodemographic aspects of patients with rapid-cycling bipolar disorder :

Our work has sought to identify sociodemographic features in patients with CRBT. This work was carried out by means of a comparison with another clinical population: patients being monitored for bipolar disorder.

The mean age at the time of our study was 41.08 years in patients with rapid cycles and 42.67 years in patients without rapid cycles. This is within the range reported in the literature. Some studies, such as those by Kato et al [18], Cruz et al [19] and Schneck et al [20] found a lower mean age in patients with rapid cycles, whereas the difference was not statistically significant in other studies, such as those by Azorin et al [14], Buoli et al [21] and Gigante et al [22].

In a 2015 study of 1225 patients by Erol et al [23], the risk of developing TBCR was higher in female patients (OR= 1.36, p = 0.009). This predominance of women in CRBT patients has been found by several authors, including Kato et al [18], Cruz et al [19] and Kupka et al [24]. Some explain this by the greater prevalence of thyroid pathologies in women [25], or by the effect of steroid hormones [26]. Others suggest that women, being at greater risk of developing depressive episodes and more likely to seek treatment for their depression, may be diagnosed with rapid cycles more frequently, due to the rapid cycle-inducing effect of antidepressants [27]. In our work, we noted no difference between the sexes in the two groups. This result is in line with that of authors such as Azorin et al [14], Gigante et al [22] and Schneck et al [20] who did not find significant differences between the sexes.

Comparisons of patients' education levels and marital status in our study did not reveal any significant differences between the TBCR and TBNCR groups. These same findings have been reported in the literature [14,19-21]. On the other hand, occupational inactivity was more frequently found in patients with rapid cycles, reflecting the alteration in their occupational functioning and, more generally, the major impact on global functioning of this progressive modality of bipolar disorder [18].

Comparison of family antecedents revealed a greater prevalence of mood disorders and substance use disorders in the relatives of TBCR patients, but this difference was not statistically significant. In the literature, several studies have demonstrated an association between the development of rapid cycles and the existence of a family history of depressive [21] or bipolar [28] mood disorders, or anxiety disorders such as panic disorder [29]. According to Fisfalen et al, the development of rapid cycles is the marker of a family trait and this progressive form of bipolarity is the expression of a greater predisposition to the development of mental disorders [30].

With regard to personal somatic antecedents, several studies assert that rapid cycles are an evolutionary modality characterised by more marked biological abnormalities [21]. Patients suffering from CRBT are thought to have greater oxidative stress and greater susceptibility to thyroid pathologies and insulin resistance [31]. In their 2014 systematic review, Carvalho et al found that the presence of rapid cycling was more often associated with thyroid comorbidity [11] despite the ongoing controversy regarding the role of thyroid hormones in this disorder [32]. Indeed, it is not yet clear whether hypothyroidism is linked to a susceptibility to CRBD or whether it is rather masked by treatments such as lithium or atypical antipsychotics [33]. Gyulai et al noted that CRBT is associated with masked hypofunction of the hypothalamic-pituitary-thyroid axis, which becomes apparent after brief treatment with lithium. They found an increased response to TRH testing in patients with rapid cycling who received a four-week course of lithium [34]. A study by Valle et al failed to find any difference in thyroid function between patients with and without rapid cycling who had not been treated with lithium or carbamazepine [35].

In our work, we found no significant difference between the antecedents of thyroid pathology in the two groups. This result is also found in the work of Kupka et al [24] and Gigante et al [22]. In our study, this may be explained by the absence of a systematic search for dysthyroidism in patients followed for bipolar disorder.

Similarly, although obesity and diabetes have been suggested as factors associated with the presence of rapid cycles [31], controversy persists as to whether these are true comorbidities or secondary effects of the treatment received. Our work, like that of Cruz et al [19] or Gigante et al [22], did not find any significant links between obesity and diabetes and the presence of rapid cycles.

In terms of substance use habits, patients with rapid cycles in our series showed a greater prevalence of alcohol and cannabis use than patients without rapid cycles. However, this difference was not statistically significant.

The prevalence of substance use disorders in bipolar patients is estimated at between 30% and 40% [36]. This use has a negative effect on the course of

bipolar disorder, with fewer periods of remission [37] and more hospitalisations [38].

Several authors have reported an association between the consumption of alcohol [30,39], cannabis [40] and other psychoactive substances and the recurrence of thymic episodes. In fact, in subjects who are vulnerable to the destabilising properties of alcohol and drugs, depressive or manic episodes may be induced. Similarly, patients with a high frequency of cycles may increase their use of substances [24]. However, while the association between the emergence of rapid cycles and alcohol abuse has been found in some studies [19,41,42], there is less agreement about the relationship with substance abuse [43].

A statistically significant increase in the use of psychotropic drugs was noted in the TBCR patients in our study. This finding may reflect a sampling effect. Psychotropic drugs are a preferred addictive substance for people suffering from addictive behaviours [44] and for patients in hospital [45], for whom access to these substances may be facilitated by their proximity to care facilities.

Among the personal antecedents reported in the literature, maltreatment and sexual abuse are found preferentially in CRBT [46]. Such abuse and maltreatment are indicators of poor emotional balance [47]. They may lead to earlier onset of mood disorders and the appearance of rapid cycles due to a greater propensity for impulsivity and emotional instability [48]. In their study, Marwaha et al noted that the risk of developing rapid cycling was 1.75 times greater in patients who had been abused as children [49]. In our study, we found a greater prevalence of previous exposure to abuse or maltreatment in TBCR patients, although this difference was not statistically significant. These results could be explained by the retrospective nature of our work.

Patients with rapid cycling in our series had significantly more personal antecedents of self-mutilation or tattooing. This phenomenon, whose prevalence in the clinical population is estimated at 21% [50], is associated in the literature with the presence of borderline or antisocial personality traits.

[51]. Mood disorders, particularly depression, have also been identified as factors associated with these behaviours [52]. Self-harm was also predictive of a greater risk of suicide attempts [53]. Personality disorders underlying mood disorders may underlie both self-harm and greater mood instability.

4. Clinical aspects of rapid-cycling bipolar disorder

Bipolar disorder with rapid cycles is clinically defined. It refers to the occurrence of a certain number of characteristic symptoms occurring on a recurrent basis. In our work, we have attempted to identify the clinical and developmental features that characterise this disorder.

4.1. Diagnostic features

To determine the diagnostic features of CRBT, we examined the type of bipolar disorder, the age of onset of the index episode and its polarities, the number of thymic episodes and hospitalisations, and the dominant polarities. This enabled us to identify certain characteristics.

Questions remain as to the correlation between the type of bipolar disorder and the risk of developing rapid cycles, especially when the sex of patients is taken into account [11]. Several older studies [54-57] and more recent ones [23,58,59] have found a greater occurrence of rapid cycles in patients with type 2 bipolar disorder. Other studies have failed to establish a significant association with subtype [60-62]. This inconsistent association could be explained by the heterogeneity of the different studies, the criteria used to define the subtypes of bipolar disorder, or the different definitions of rapid cycling used by different authors [20]. In our study, only two patients were diagnosed with type 2 bipolar disorder. No association was therefore established between the subtype of the disorder and the appearance of rapid cycles.

The under-representation of patients treated for type 2 bipolar disorder has been encountered in other studies of bipolarity in Tunisia [63]. The explanation put forward is that patients are most frequently hospitalised for initial manic episodes and are consequently diagnosed with bipolar disorder type 1. Fewer are hospitalised for depressive episodes. The result is a lower number of bipolar type 2 disorders [64].

With regard to index episodes, patients with rapid cycles in our series had an age of onset of disorders 2.29 years younger than patients without rapid cycles (although this difference was not statistically significant). In TBCR patients, the index episode was more often depressive in nature. This earlier onset of bipolar disorder has been consistently reported in the literature [18,32,65,66]. Many authors agree that the onset of the illness at a younger age is an important predictive factor for the recurrence of thymic episodes [22]. Thus, Schneck et al, in a prospective cohort study of bipolar patients, identified two types of patients according to the course of their illness [62]. The first group consists of patients who begin their disorder at around 20 years of age and who have a more stable course of the disorder with a lower rate of recurrence. A second group consists of those who have a less stable course and who begin their disorder approximately three years earlier, in mid-adolescence. Some authors, such as Ernst et al [67] and Post et al [68], suggest the role of an "ignition" or "kindling" mechanism in the early onset of bipolar disorder, which induces a recurrence of thymic episodes in this type of patient, without the need for triggering factors. However, this phenomenon remains poorly explained, because although the majority of studies emphasise the relationship between early age of onset and recurrence of thymic episodes, the association with the development of rapid cycles is not always established [62,69,70].

In several international and local studies, depressive polarities during the first thymic episode have been noted more frequently in patients with rapid cycles [71-73]. Thus, in a Tunisian study, Bram et al found that the subsequent development of rapid cycles was found in patients who had had a thymic episode with depressive polarities [74]. However, other authors, who had not demonstrated this association [22,70], suggested instead the role of antidepressant treatment during the first episode [20].

With regard to the recurrence of episodes, our results - which noted a greater number of thymic episodes, a greater number of manic episodes and depressive episodes, and a greater number of hospital admissions in patients with rapid cycles - are consistent with the literature. Indeed, several retrospective and prospective studies agree in associating the presence of rapid cycles with a greater number of characteristic manic or depressive thymic episodes over a lifetime [11,14,18,24]. These results emphasise that the passage into rapid cycles corresponds more to a perennial mode of evolution of the disorder than to a transient evolutionary accident.

For hypomanic episodes, studies are less concordant: a higher frequency in TBCR patients has been noted by some authors [20,21] whereas in other studies the difference between patients with and without rapid cycles was not significant. In our study, the mean number of hypomanic episodes was 0.38 and 0.30 episodes per patient, respectively. This low number could be explained by the tolerance of a relatively mild thymic symptomatology in the Tunisian sociocultural context, which results in underdiagnosis of this type of episode [63,75].

Similarly, the higher number of hospitalisations in patients with CRBT has been reported by several authors, including Azorin et al [14] and Kupka et al [24]. In a recent study, Buoli et al emphasise the higher number of hospitalisations in the year preceding the onset of rapid cycles [21]. Authors such as Serretti et al found no difference in the number of hospitalisations between patients with and without rapid cycles. They explain this discrepancy in results by the difference in management and the capacity of care facilities [70].

With regard to dominant polarity, several authors have demonstrated the association between a dominant depressive polarity - present in more than two-thirds of episodes - and the presence of rapid cycles [32,76]. Calabrese et al even describe depression as a specific marker of rapid cycling [13] and suggest that antidepressant prescription is a potential source of induction of these rapid-cycling forms. Our results are consistent with these findings. However, other authors such as Buoli et al or Gigante et al have not found this predominant depressive polarity in their studies [21,22].

4.2. Clinical characteristics of thymic episodes

In our series, patients with CRBT had significantly more melancholic features than patients without rapid cycling. There were no statistically significant differences in other clinical features. In the literature, the main clinical feature that stands out in most studies is the greater severity of depressive episodes in patients with CRBT. Coryell et al have suggested the presence of greater depressive morbidity [61] and Schneck et al have emphasised that depression is more severe, especially in patients with type 2 bipolar disorder [20]. This severity remains to be interpreted taking into account a potential selection bias.

The psychotic characteristics of thymic episodes in TBCR patients were not as unanimously emphasised by the authors. While the work of Buoli et al [21] and Kato et al [18] found a greater prevalence of psychotic elements in patients with rapid cycles, other studies such as Cruz et al and Schneck et al found no difference [19,62] or more psychotic elements in patients without rapid cycles [14]. Haro et al noted that rapid cycles were less present in the psychotic form of mania [77]. According to these authors, rapid cycles and psychotic features are independent pathological mechanisms that mark severity in bipolar disorder. Thus, morbidity in rapid cycles would be more related to an emotional dimension than to a psychotic dimension [20].

4.3. Associated psychiatric disorders

In our work, patients with rapid cycling were more likely to have psychiatric comorbidities than patients without rapid cycling. No prevalence of a psychiatric disorder compared separately showed a significant difference despite a greater frequency in the TBCR group for cannabis use disorder and personality disorders. Substance use disorder, alcohol use disorder and cannabis use disorder are frequently cited as comorbidities preferentially associated with the presence of rapid cycling [21,24,78]. However, this result was not found in the meta-analysis by Valenti et al [43]. This disparity in results could be explained by the heterogeneity of the samples and the differences in the inclusion criteria used [14].

An associated pathological personality has also been suggested by several authors [18,79,80]. These personality disorders often present diagnostic difficulties in distinguishing rapid cycles from the mood instability seen, for example, in borderline personality disorder, especially as frequent substance use sustains thymic fluctuations [7].

Other psychiatric comorbidities have been found in studies such as anxiety disorders [24], neurodevelopmental disorders [18] and eating disorders [21].

4.4. Suicide attempts

Our results showed a higher prevalence of suicide attempts in patients with rapid cycles. This suicidal dimension as a prognostic marker has received particular attention in studies of bipolar disorder [81]. Carvalho et al, in a review of the literature, highlighted a greater suicidal dimension in patients with rapid cycles [11]. This characteristic, which has a high prognostic value, was present in various studies [22,43,82,83] and some authors emphasise a higher number of suicide attempts in these patients [19,21,22].

Depressive polarity has been cited as an incriminating factor [84]. Similarly, the long duration of the disease, due to its early onset, is thought to be associated with heavy demands on the central nervous system, leading to a reorganisation marked by increased vulnerability to stress factors. These changes worsen the overall prognosis and facilitate suicide attempts [85,86].

5. Therapeutic aspects of rapid-cycling bipolar disorder

Between induction facilitated by possible iatrogenicity and recurrence of thymic relapses requiring the use of drug combinations, the therapeutic aspects of CRBT represent a major challenge in understanding and managing this progressive condition.

The role of antidepressants in the onset of rapid cycling has long been debated. Since the role of tricyclic antidepressants in the onset of rapid cycling was described in 1979 by Wehr et al [16], several authors have emphasised the association between this evolutionary mode and the prescription of antidepressants. Thus, according to Schneck et al [20], the probability of developing rapid cycles increases linearly with the use of antidepressants: patients on this type of treatment have three times the risk of developing rapid cycles compared with patients who do not use them. Antidepressants therefore appear to have a potentiating effect on the development and aggravation of rapid cycling [87]. However, for Schneck et al, the causal relationship cannot be accepted despite this statistical association [62]. While several studies have highlighted the negative impact of antidepressant prescription on the induction of rapid cycles, others have not found the same results. Coryell et al explain this association by a non-causal relationship. This association is thought to be secondary to the presence of a dominant depressive polarity associated with rapid cycling rather than to the direct effect of antidepressants [61]. In our work, we found a statistically significant association between the use of serotonin reuptake inhibitor antidepressants and the presence of rapid cycling. This association was not significant for tricyclic antidepressants despite a higher prevalence of use in TBCR patients. This lack of statistical association should be put into perspective, given the small number of patients on this treatment in our series.

Dunner's identification and definition of rapid cycling as an evolving modality in bipolar disorder was initiated by his study of the failure of lithium treatment in a patient population [8]. This particular therapeutic feature was subsequently found in various studies [21,66]. In their analysis of the results of 16 studies looking at the effect of rapid cycling and different therapeutic choices on the outcome of patients with bipolar disorder, Tondo et al noted that rapid cycling was associated with a poor response to treatment [88]. The authors also noted a certain equivalence in the efficacy of mood stabilisers in patients with rapid cycles [22,89]. For Fountoulakis et al, lithium and sodium valproate had comparable effects and both showed low efficacy [90].

In our work, we did not note any significant differences in the thymoregulators prescribed and received in the two groups of patients.

In our series, four out of five patients with rapid cycling were treated with atypical antipsychotics. The same proportion was treated with conventional antipsychotics. The difference with patients without rapid cycling was not significant. In the literature, conventional and atypical antipsychotics had comparable effects in patients with and without rapid cycling [21,22]. Certain molecules such as olanzapine, aripiprazole or quetiapine had shown efficacy in the acute phases in patients with CRBD. Olanzapine had a comparable effect to antiepileptics such as divalproate [90,91]. The efficacy of risperidone or clozapine has not been demonstrated [62]. According to Fountoulakis et al, the use of atypical antipsychotics in maintenance treatment has shown "promising results which remain to be confirmed" [90].

With regard to sedatives, the prescription of benzodiazepines was equivalent between the two groups. However, a higher prescription of hypnotics such as antihistamines and zolpidem was found in patients with rapid cycles. Antihistamine hypnotics and zolpidem represent a therapeutic recourse for patients with more severe symptoms and a partial response to treatment.

6. Course and prognosis of rapid-cycling bipolar disorder

There is almost unanimous agreement in the literature that there are negative prognostic factors associated with CRBT. The severity of this disorder and its impact on patients' overall functioning are thought to be linked to the long duration of the illness, particularly the depressive phase. Patients with rapid cycles have a longer lifetime depressive phase than other patients with bipolar disorder [19,24].

TBCR patients have more occupational dysfunction [19] and more functional disability [18,19]. For Kato et al, the time spent in relapse has a negative impact on the cognitive abilities and quality of life of patients with rapid cycles [18]. In this context, a higher prevalence of occupational inactivity was noted in the TBCR patients in our study. For Kessing et al, the increasing number of thymic episodes seems to be associated with an increased risk of relapse, an increase in the duration of episodes, a worsening of symptomatology, a reduction in the threshold for episode development and an increase in the risk of developing dementia [92]. Thus, the emergence of rapid cycles in patients with bipolar disorder modifies the functional prognosis and disrupts quality of life in the long term. Rapid cycling may also have a more immediate impact, notably through addictive comorbidity and increased suicidal risk [18].

From an evolutionary point of view, some authors place the occurrence of rapid cycles within a course of the illness marked by early onset and long course. Rapid cycles are thought to reflect a long course of bipolar disorder that began during adolescence or even childhood [93]. The reduction in the duration of free intervals and the absence of individualisable triggers for thymic episodes are thought to be precursors of a sensitisation process leading to the occurrence of rapid cycles [14]. This evolutionary pattern would therefore be a marker of recurrence and resistance to treatment, indicating an advanced stage of the disease [21]. However, rapid cycles could be a transient phenomenon, as emphasised by certain studies [20,65]. It therefore calls for particular vigilance and meticulous clinical monitoring to ensure better compliance with treatment and prevent costs in terms of inactivity and the number of hospital admissions, as well as complications such as addictive and suicidal behaviour.

7. The concept of rapid cycles: an ancient notion under permanent reconstruction

The French authors Jean-Pierre and Jules Falret, Ballet and Marce reported from the 1850s on recurrent forms of madness with rapid inversion that could be preceded by a circular or remittent evolution (i.e. without a free interval) [94]. In the 1880s, Jules Baillarget and then his pupil Antoine Ritti provided the first clinical descriptions, speaking of much shorter episodes of double-form madness in which the two periods did not extend beyond six to eight days [95], or of circular double-form madness with a three-day period [96]. Lastly, Kraepelin was responsible for the descriptions of manic-depressive madness in Anglo-Saxon works [97].

The term "rapid cycling" was first introduced in 1974 by Dunner and Fieve to describe a group of patients with a poor response to lithium salts in whom they recorded a high frequency of cycles [8]. The number of four or more thymic episodes per year was determined arbitrarily in order to have a large population of patients to study [98]. This initial definition was then taken up and introduced into the DSM-IV [9] as a clinical specificity for bipolar disorder type 1 and type 2.

Other ultra-rapid forms with more than eight episodes per year have been described, including daily thymic inversion and ultradian forms where the cycle is less than 24 hours [99]. However, these ultra-rapid forms have not been included in the DSM.

The rapid cycle can therefore be conceptualised in different ways: as a high frequency of separate episodes which may be of any polarity, or as a temporal sequence of episodes of opposite polarity [69,100].

For their 1974 definition, Dunner and Fieve opted for a simple approach consisting of counting each thymic episode, regardless of its polarity, taking into account criteria of duration and severity, and then delimiting a cut-off point of four episodes per year [98]. This is also the approach adopted by the DSM and the definition we have chosen for our work.

Thus, the thymic episode is classified by the number of symptoms and by its duration. The minimum duration is one week for a manic episode, four days for a hypomanic episode and two weeks for a typical depressive episode.

The choice of the number of episodes required to define the rapid cycle may seem arbitrary. However, some studies, such as the multicentre study by Baeur et al, have highlighted the operational nature of this choice [69]. Thus, this approach would have made it possible to consider the evolutionary aspects of CRBT and to go beyond the purely descriptive aspect of definitions based on alternating episodes of opposite polarities [101].

Other authors have tried to propose alternative definitions for rapid cycling. In their 1999 study, Maj et al used four different definitions by modifying the criteria of duration and severity of symptoms. They found that the DSM definition, although reliable, did not cover the full spectrum of rapid cycling [100].

In this respect, more recent studies have focused on a dimensional approach, considering the rapid cycle as a continuum between two extremes: the absence of thymic episodes and the continuous disorder (with persistence of signs between periods of exacerbation) [24]. Thus, these studies have demonstrated statistical links between the number of thymic episodes and the clinical characteristics observed, by adopting a qualitative approach rather than the conventional quantitative approach. However, they were unable to propose a better threshold for defining rapid cycles [24,30].

At the extreme end of this frequency continuum are the ultrafast and ultradian cycles that do not meet the DSM criteria for bipolar disorder type 1 and type 2. The high proportion of patients who do not meet the criteria for the duration of free intervals or of the episodes themselves have been grouped together as bipolar disorders not *otherwise specified* (NOS) in the DSM. It might be judicious to add specification with rapid cycles to this category, as proposed by Bauer et al [101].

In the same sense, cyclothymia would be considered part of this continuum if the severity of symptoms were removed. This approach would make it possible to include a new category of patients in studies of rapid cycling and to broaden the spectrum of this disorder [102].

8. Recommendations

Our study highlighted a number of diagnostic and clinical features that help to define the clinical profile of patients suffering from CRBT.

The identification of patients with rapid cycles or at risk of developing them requires a meticulous history to search for all the thymic episodes presented by the patients. It therefore seems essential to estimate the rate of thymic recurrence for each patient, taking into account pauci-symptomatic episodes.

- The depressive index episode and its onset at a young age are elements that should alert the clinician. Similarly, certain behaviours have been described in patients with rapid cycles, notably the presence of self-mutilation or tattoos and the use of psychoactive substances. The presence of such factors calls for therapeutic vigilance and enhanced thymoregulation.

- The occurrence of rapid cycles is a major risk factor for suicide. This requires close clinical monitoring of patients and optimisation of treatment.

- The use of antidepressants is associated with the appearance of rapid cycles in most of the literature, as well as in our work. Their use in the treatment of bipolar depression must therefore be carefully considered and well supervised. In patients with rapid cycles, the use of antidepressants is not recommended [103,104]. Antidepressants are thought to play a role in destabilising patients, even those on associated thymoregulatory therapy.

- When monitoring patients with bipolar disorder, hormone assays to look for dyshyroidism should be carried out as a matter of course.

- Rigorous psychoeducation of the patient and those around him is also essential in order to detect any changes in symptomatology and prevent mood swings.

- The first step in treatment is to prevent the onset of this progressive course. This prevention involves screening populations at risk and avoiding treatments likely to induce this transition.

- CRBT is a progressive modality, the management of which is often made difficult by the inadequate therapeutic response to thymoregulators, particularly lithium. Treatment in the acute phase is based on the prescription of atypical antipsychotics such as quetiapine, olanzapine or aripiprazole. Maintenance treatment is often based on a combination of several mood regulators [90,104]. Reducing the rate of recurrence should be the main therapeutic objective, with specific, personalised management in specialised settings.

- The reinforcement of thymoregulatory treatments must be integrated into a bio-psycho-social approach. The population of patients treated for CRBT is particularly vulnerable to unemployment. More sustained attempts at socio-professional reintegration are indicated for these patients.

V. CONCLUSIONS

Bipolar disorder is a frequent and particularly severe psychiatric pathology that causes significant morbidity and mortality. It presents in heterogeneous clinical forms in terms of expression, course, response to treatment and associated comorbidities.

The rapid cycles introduced in 1974 by Dunner and Fieve in their work with patients showing a poor response to lithium salts have been adopted as a clinical specification for bipolar disorder type 1 and type 2 in the DSM-IV.

They are defined, according to the DSM, by the presence over the last twelve months of at least four thymic episodes meeting the criteria of a characteristic depressive, manic or hypomanic episode. The episodes are delimited by the occurrence of a complete or partial remission lasting at least two months or by the transition to an episode of opposite polarity.

The lifetime prevalence of rapid-cycling bipolar disorder is estimated at between 25.8% and 43%. Many authors have associated this clinical form with specific clinical, therapeutic and prognostic features.

Rapid cycling bipolar disorder (RBCD) has an important prognostic aspect due to its resistance to treatment, the functional disability it causes and the addictive and suicidal comorbidities associated with it.

This evolutionary modality has not been well described in the literature. The profile of patients presenting with this clinical specification is poorly defined, and the therapeutic options are not clearly codified. Tunisian studies on this subject are rare.

In this context, we conducted a retrospective descriptive and comparative study to describe the sociodemographic, clinical and therapeutic characteristics of patients with bipolar disorder with rapid cycles, and to compare these characteristics with those of patients with bipolar disorder without rapid cycles.

Using a pre-established epidemiological and clinical form, we collected data reported in the medical records of patients admitted to psychiatric wards "A", "B" and "G" at Razi Hospital during the period 2015 to 2017 and followed for bipolar disorder for at least 2 years.

We began by investigating the sociodemographic characteristics and tracing the clinical and therapeutic history of patients since their initial thymic episode. We performed a descriptive analysis of data relating to patients with rapid cycling bipolar disorder (RBCD). We then compared these data with those relating to patients with bipolar disorder without rapid cycles (TBNCR).

Descriptive analysis of the patients with CRBT (n=37) revealed a mean age at the time of the study of 41.08 years, with a sex ratio of 2.08. Three-quarters of the patients lived in urban areas and more than half lived in Greater Tunis. Three quarters of the patients lived in urban areas and more than half lived in Greater Tunis. Parental consanguinity was found in 27% of patients, parental divorce in 10.8% and the death of at least one parent in 40.5%.

Almost half of the patients had secondary education, and around a third had primary education. One patient in six had vocational training.

97.3% of TBCR patients were occupationally inactive. They lived on average incomes (73%) and low incomes (18.9%). Single people accounted for 48.6% of patients, married 40.5% and divorced 10.8%. The majority (94.6%) lived with a close relative.

The most common family psychiatric antecedent was mood disorder in 43.2% of patients, followed by psychotic disorder in 18.9% and substance use disorder in 10.8%. A family antecedent of anxiety disorder was found in 8.1% of patients and a family antecedent of suicide attempt in 8.1%.

In terms of personal history, six out of ten patients with TBCR regularly consumed alcohol. More than a third used cannabis and more than a quarter psychotropic drugs. Volatile solvents were used by 5.4% of patients and amphetamines by 2.7%. None of the patients had injected drugs. Self-mutilation or tattoos were found in 27% of patients and a history of incarceration or arrest in 29.7%. A personal history of abuse was found in 21.6% of patients and sexual abuse in 8.1%.

The TBCR patients had a history of cardiovascular pathologies such as obesity in six patients, arterial hypertension and diabetes in two patients respectively. Dyslipidemia and coronary artery disease were present in one patient each. We found infectious pathologies such as tuberculosis in two patients and viral hepatitis in one patient. Dermatological pathologies such as vitiligo and psoriasis were present in one and two patients respectively.

Clinically, the vast majority of patients (94.6%) had a diagnosis of type 1 bipolar disorder. The mean age of onset of the disorder was 23.73 years, with an index episode of depressive polarity in 56.8% of cases. The mean number of thymic episodes was 13.95. The mean number of manic, depressive and hypomanic episodes was 9.35, 4.22 and 0.38 episodes respectively. The mean number of hospital admissions was 10.51, with a mean length of stay of 17.95 days. A dominantly manic polarity was found in 56.76% of cases and a dominantly depressive polarity in 27.03%. Psychotic features were noted in almost two-thirds of the thymic episodes. Atypical features, mixed features and anxiety distress were each present in 10% of episodes.

Melancholic features were noted in 8.1% of episodes.

More than half the patients had a psychiatric comorbidity. Alcohol use disorder was present in 10.8% of patients and cannabis use disorder in 21.6%. One-fifth of patients had an associated personality disorder. More than half the patients had attempted suicide, with an average of 2.16 attempts per suicidal patient.

Therapeutically, tricyclic antidepressants were prescribed in 13.5% of patients, serotonin reuptake inhibitors in 37.8% and serotonin and noradrenaline reuptake inhibitors in 8.1%.

Conventional antipsychotics and atypical antipsychotics were each used in 83.8% of patients. All patients with CRBT received anticonvulsants and 18.9% received lithium. Clozapine was used in only one patient. Benzodiazepines were prescribed for 83.8% of patients, and antihistamines and zolpidem for 56.8%. Finally, electroconvulsive therapy and transcranial magnetic stimulation were used in one and three patients respectively.

A comparative study of socio-demographic data and antecedents revealed a significantly higher rate of occupational inactivity among TBCR patients, a greater prevalence of self-mutilation and tattoos, and a higher frequency of psychotropic drug use. Alcohol and cannabis use were more frequent in this group, although the difference with TBNCR patients was not statistically significant. Comparison of the other sociodemographic parameters did not reveal any significant differences.

Clinically, the comparative study found that the mean age of onset of the disease was 2.29 years earlier in TBCR patients. Patients in this group had an index episode of depressive polarity and a dominant depressive polarity significantly more frequently. They had a significantly higher number of thymic, manic and depressive episodes and hospitalisations than TBNCR patients, and were significantly more likely to have melancholic features.

In terms of therapy, a significantly higher proportion of patients with CRBT had received treatment with serotonin reuptake inhibitors and hypnotics such as antihistamines and zolpidem. The use of tricyclic antidepressants was more common in CRBT patients, but the difference with NNRBT patients was not significant.

The originality and interest of our study was to describe a profile of patients presenting with a rarely individualised form of bipolar disorder. In fact, this work, which was both descriptive and comparative, shed light on a population that has been little studied in Tunisian studies. It retraced the long and heterogeneous course of these patients, highlighting specific therapeutic and prognostic issues. Our work has methodological limitations due to the relatively small size of the population and the retrospective nature of the study. Recall and selection biases therefore had to be taken into account when interpreting our results.

On the basis of the data collected and bibliographic research, it would appear that depressive symptomatology is an indicator of CRBT. A predominantly depressive symptomatology is an element whose presence should alert us to the propensity to develop this progressive form.

In the same sense, an index episode of depressive polarity - especially at a relatively young age - and a dominant depressive polarity prompt careful monitoring of patients with bipolar disorder to detect accelerated cycles. Particular attention should be paid if antidepressant treatment has been used. Although tricyclic antidepressants have been implicated in cycle acceleration in several studies, our results show that selective serotonin reuptake inhibitors are also associated with the occurrence of rapid cycles.

Our work has enabled us to identify a number of behaviours associated with CRBT. Tattoos and self-mutilation, consumption of psychotropic drugs and other substances such as alcohol and cannabis should raise the alarm and prompt surveillance.

CRBT is a severe evolutionary modality in terms of its clinical expression. Our results have highlighted the significant morbidity associated with it, as evidenced by the large number of thymic relapses, the high number of hospitalisations and the negative impact on professional activity. The severity of thymic episodes, particularly the greater frequency of melancholic features, and the higher prevalence of suicide attempts are important prognostic factors.

In our work, rapid cycling has been associated with greater psychiatric comorbidity, which should be investigated. Thus, a substance use disorder or a personality disorder may have a negative influence on the prognosis of these patients.

In the light of these results, we propose the following recommendations to optimise the management of patients at risk of developing CRBT and, even more so, those who already have CRBT.

A careful history to search for all previous thymic episodes and a good estimate of the rate of thymic recurrence, taking into account pauci-symptomatic episodes, are essential to identify patients with rapid cycles or at risk of developing them. Certain behaviours have been described in patients with rapid cycles, notably the presence of self-mutilation or tattoos and the use of psychoactive substances. Similarly, the depressive index episode and its onset at a young age are elements that can alert the clinician and encourage therapeutic vigilance with more vigorous thymoregulation.

The occurrence of rapid cycles is a major risk factor for suicide, requiring close clinical monitoring of patients and optimisation of both pharmacological and psychotherapeutic treatment.

The use of antidepressants in the treatment of bipolar depression should be avoided.

Patients with bipolar disorder should be monitored systematically for the presence of thyroid dysfunction. Rigorous psychoeducation of the patient and those around him is also essential, in order to detect any change in symptomatology and prevent mood swings.

The first step in treating CRBT is to prevent its onset by screening at-risk populations and avoiding treatments likely to induce this transition. The management of CRBT is often made difficult by the inadequate therapeutic response to thymoregulators, particularly lithium. Atypical antipsychotics such as quetiapine, olanzapine or aripiprazole are useful in the acute phase. Maintenance treatment is often based on a combination of several mood regulators.

In CRBT, the main therapeutic objective should be to reduce the rate of recurrence, with specific, personalised treatment in specialised settings. The reinforcement of mood-regulating treatments must be integrated into a bio-psycho-social approach. The population of patients treated for CRBT is particularly vulnerable to unemployment. More sustained attempts at socio-professional reintegration are indicated for these patients.

In conclusion, CRBT is a relatively common progressive modality. It is associated with depressive and suicidal aspects, making it an important prognostic issue. Prevention of its development involves early detection of patients at risk, rationalisation of the use of antidepressants in bipolar depression, prevention of addictive comorbidities and optimisation of thymoregulatory treatment.

There is still much debate about the place of rapid cycling in the evolutionary history of bipolar disorder. Classical categorical considerations are increasingly giving way to a dimensional approach which places cyclicity at the centre of a continuum of frequency, where cycles constitute a form oscillating between the absence of thymic episodes and a disorder of continuous appearance with persistence of signs between periods of exacerbation. Prospective studies could refine the profile of patients with rapid cycles and provide more information on the repercussions of this form of the disorder.

VI. REFERENCES

1.   Judd LL, Akiskal HS, Schettler PJ, Endicott J, Maser J, Solomon DA, et al. The longterm natural history of the weekly symptomatic status of bipolar I disorder. Arch Gen Psychiatry. 2002 Jun;59(6):530-7.

2.   Rosa AR, Gonzalez-Ortega I, Gonzalez-Pinto A, Echeburua E, Comes M, Martinez-Aran A, et al. One-year psychosocial functioning in patients in the early vs. late stage of bipolar disorder. Acta Psychiatr Scand. 2012 Apr;125(4):335–41.

3.   Haustgen T, Akiskal H. French antecedents of "contemporary" concepts in the American Psychiatric Association's classification of bipolar (mood) disorders. J Affect Disord. 2006 Dec;96(3):149–63.

4.   Crocq MA. Chapter 1: Manic-depressive and bipolar disorders: History of the concept. In: Bourgeois ML. Les troubles bipolaires. Cachan: Lavoisier; 2014. p.3-9.

5.   Ernoul A, Mouseler A, Dubois de Prisque G, Poussevin C, Roquelaure Y, Duverger P, et al. Consideration critique sur I'extension de la bipolarite, psychopathologie des mouvements d'humeur et de l'euphorie morbide. Ann Med Psychol. Oct 2014;172(8):599–605.

6.   Merikangas KR, Jin R, He JP, Kessler RC, Lee S, Sampson NA, et al. Prevalence and correlates of bipolar spectrum disorder in the world mental health survey initiative. Arch Gen Psychiatry. 2011 Mar;68(3):241–51.

7.   Gay C, Masson M, Bellivier F. Chapter 28. Rapid cycling bipolar disorder. In: Bourgeois ML. Les troubles bipolaires. Cachan: Lavoisier; 2014. p.205–13.

8.   Dunner DL, Fieve RR. Clinical factors in lithium carbonate prophylaxis failure. Arch Gen Psychiatry. 1974 Feb;30(2):229–33.

9.   Association AP. Diagnostic and statistical manual of mental disorders: DSM-IV. Washington: American Psychiatric Association; 1994.

10. Association AP. Diagnostic and statistical manual of mental disorders: DSM-5. American Psychiatric Association; 2013.

11. Carvalho AF, Dimellis D, Gonda X, Vieta E, McIntyre RS, Fountoulakis KN. Rapid cycling in bipolar disorder: A systematic review. J Clin Psychiatry. 2014 Jun;75(6):578-86.

12. Alarcon RD. Rapid cycling affective disorders: A clinical review. Compr Psychiatry. 1985 Nov;26(6):522–40.

13. Calabrese JR, Shelton MD, Bowden CL, Rapport DJ, Suppes T, Shirley ER, et al. Bipolar rapid cycling: Focus on depression as its hallmark. J Clin Psychiatry. 2001;62 Suppl 14:34–41.

14. Azorin J-M, Kaladjian A, Adida M, Hantouche EG, Hameg A, Lancrenon S, et al. Factors associated with rapid cycling in bipolar I manic patients: Findings from a French national study. CNS Spectr. 2008 Sep;13(9):780–7.

15. Feinman JA, Dunner DL. The effect of alcohol and substance abuse on the course of bipolar affective disorder. J Affect Disord. 1996 Feb;37(1):43–9.

16. Wehr TA, Goodwin FK. Rapid cycling in manic-depressives induced by tricyclic antidepressants. Arch Gen Psychiatry. 1979 May;36(5):555–9.

17. Colom F, Vieta E, Daban C, Pacchiarotti I, Sanchez-Moreno J. Clinical and therapeutic implications of predominant polarity in bipolar disorder. J Affect Disord. 2006 Jul;93(1):13–7.

18. Kato M, Adachi N, Kubota Y, Azekawa T, Ueda H, Edagawa K, et al. Clinical features related to rapid cycling and one-year euthymia in bipolar disorder patients: A multicenter treatment survey for bipolar disorder in psychiatric clinics. J Psychiatr Res. 2020 Dec;131:228–34.

19. Cruz N, Vieta E, Comes M, Haro JM, Reed C, Bertsch J, et al. Rapid-cycling bipolar I disorder: Course and treatment outcome of a large sample across Europe. J Psychiatr Res. 2008 Oct;42(13):1068–75.

20. Schneck CD, Miklowitz DJ, Calabrese JR, Allen MH, Thomas MR, Wisniewski SR, et al. Phenomenology of rapid-cycling bipolar disorder: Data from the first 500 participants in the Systematic Treatment Enhancement Program. Am J Psychiatry. 2004 Oct;161(10):1902–8.

21. Buoli M, Cesana BM, Maina G, Conca A, Fagiolini A, Steardo L, et al. Correlates of current rapid-cycling bipolar disorder: Results from the Italian multicentric RENDiBi study. Eur Psychiatry J. 2019 Oct;62:82–9.

22. Gigante AD, Barenboim IY, Dias R, Toniolo RA, Mendonca T, Miranda-Scippa A, et al. Psychiatric and clinical correlates of rapid cycling bipolar disorder: A cross-sectional study. Braz J Psychiatry. 2016 Jun;38(4):270–4.

23. Erol A, Winham SJ, McElroy SL, Frye MA, Prieto ML, Cuellar-Barboza AB, et al. Sex differences in the risk of rapid cycling and other indicators of adverse illness course in patients with bipolar I and II disorder. Bipolar Disord. 2015 Sep;17(6):670-6.

24. Kupka RW, Luckenbaugh DA, Post RM, Suppes T, Altshuler LL, Keck PE, et al. Comparison of rapid-cycling and non-rapid-cycling bipolar disorder based on prospective mood ratings in 539 outpatients. Am J Psychiatry. 2005 Jul;162(7):1273-80.

25. Cowdry RW, Wehr TA, Zis AP, Goodwin FK. Thyroid abnormalities associated with rapid-cycling bipolar illness. Arch Gen Psychiatry. 1983 Apr;40(4):414-20.

26. Price WA, DiMarzio L. Premenstrual tension syndrome in rapid-cycling bipolar affective disorder. J Clin Psychiatry. 1986 Aug;47(8):415-7.

27. Calabrese JR, Shelton MD, Rapport DJ, Kujawa M, Kimmel SE, Caban S. Current research on rapid cycling bipolar disorder and its treatment. J Affect Disord. 2001 Dec;67(1):241-55.

28. Vieta E, Panicali F, Goetz I, Reed C, Comes M, Tohen M. Olanzapine monotherapy and olanzapine combination therapy in the treatment of mania: 12-week results from the European Mania in Bipolar Longitudinal Evaluation of Medication (EMBLEM) observational study. J Affect Disord. 2008 Feb;106(1):63-72.

29. MacKinnon DF, Zandi PP, Gershon ES, Nurnberger JI, DePaulo JR. Association of rapid mood switching with panic disorder and familial panic risk in familial bipolar disorder. Am J Psychiatry. 2003 Sep;160(9):1696-8.

30. Fisfalen ME, Schulze TG, DePaulo JR, DeGroot LJ, Badner JA, McMahon FJ. Familial variation in episode frequency in bipolar affective disorder. Am J Psychiatry. 2005 Jul;162(7):1266-72.

31. Buoli M, Serati M, Altamura AC. Biological aspects and candidate biomarkers for rapidcycling in bipolar disorder: A systematic review. Psychiatry Res. 2017 Dec;258:565-75.

32. Lee S, Tsang A, Kessler RC, Jin R, Sampson N, Andrade L, et al. Rapid-cycling bipolar disorder: Cross-national community study. Br J Psychiatry. 2010 Mar;196(3):217-25.

33. Buoli M, Serati M, Altamura AC. Is the combination of a mood stabilizer plus an antipsychotic more effective than mono-therapies in long-term treatment of bipolar disorder? A systematic review. J Affect Disord. 2014 Jan;152:12-8.

34. Gyulai L, Bauer M, Bauer MS, Garda-Espana F, Cnaan A, Whybrow PC. Thyroid hypofunction in patients with rapid-cycling bipolar disorder after lithium challenge. Biol Psychiatry. 2003 May;53(10):899-905.

35. Valle J, Ayuso-Gutierrez JL, Abril A, Ayuso-Mateos JL. Evaluation of thyroid function in lithium-naive bipolar patients. Eur Psychiatry. 1999 Oct;14(6):341-5.

36. Hunt GE, Malhi GS, Cleary M, Lai HMX, Sitharthan T. Prevalence of comorbid bipolar and substance use disorders in clinical settings, 1990-2015: Systematic review and meta-analysis. J Affect Disord. 2016 Dec;206:331-49.

37. Goldberg JF, Garno JL, Leon AC, Kocsis JH, Portera L. A history of substance abuse complicates remission from acute mania in bipolar disorder. J Clin Psychiatry. 1999 Nov;60(11):733-40.

38. Cassidy F, Ahearn EP, Carroll BJ. Substance abuse in bipolar disorder. Bipolar Disord. 2001 Aug;3(4):181-8.

39. Strakowski SM, DelBello MP, Fleck DE, Adler CM, Anthenelli RM, Keck PE Jr, et al. Effects of co-occurring alcohol abuse on the course of bipolar disorder following a first hospitalization for mania. Arch Gen Psychiatry. 2005 Aug;62(8):851-8.

40. Strakowski SM, DelBello MP, Fleck DE, Adler CM, Anthenelli RM, Keck PE Jr, et al. Effects of co-occurring cannabis use disorders on the course of bipolar disorder after a first hospitalization for mania. Arch Gen Psychiatry. 2007 Jan;64(1):57-64.

41. Ostacher MJ, Perlis RH, Nierenberg AA, Calabrese J, Stange JP, Salloum I, et al. Impact of substance use disorders on recovery from episodes of depression in bipolar disorder patients: Prospective data from the Systematic Treatment Enhancement Program for Bipolar Disorder (STEP-BD). Am J Psychiatry. 2010 Mar;167(3):289-97.

42. Rakofsky JJ, Dunlop BW. Do alcohol use disorders destabilize the course of bipolar disorder? J Affect Disord. 2013 Feb;145(1):1-10.

43. Valenti M, Pacchiarotti I, Undurraga J, Bonnin CM, Popovic D, Goikolea JM, et al. Risk factors for rapid cycling in bipolar disorder. Bipolar Disord. 2015 Aug;17(5):549-59.

44. Sellami R, Feki I, Zahaf A, Masmoudi J. The profile of drug users in Tunisia: Implications for prevention. Tunis Med. 2016 Sep;94(8):531-4.

45. Mustapha SB, Homri W, Labbane R. Bipolar disorder and substance use disorders in a Tunisian sample. Eur Psychiatry. 2017 Apr;41(1):466.

46. Leverich GS, McElroy SL, Suppes T, Keck PE, Denicoff KD, Nolen WA, et al. Early physical and sexual abuse associated with an adverse course of bipolar illness. Biol Psychiatry. 2002 Feb;51(4):288-97.

47. MacKinnon DF, Pies R. Affective instability as rapid cycling: Theoretical and clinical implications for borderline personality and bipolar spectrum disorders. Bipolar Disord. 2006 Feb;8(1):1-14.

48. Garno JL, Goldberg JF, Ramirez PM, Ritzler BA. Impact of childhood abuse on the clinical course of bipolar disorder. Br J Psychiatry. 2005 Feb;186(2):121-5.

49. Marwaha S, Briley PM, Perry A, Rankin P, DiFlorio A, Craddock N, et al. Explaining why childhood abuse is a risk factor for poorer clinical course in bipolar disorder: A path analysis of 923 people with bipolar I disorder. Psychol Med. 2020 Oct;50(14):2346-54.

50. Klonsky ED. The functions of deliberate self-injury: A review of the evidence. Clin Psychol Rev. 2007 Mar;27(2):226-39.

51. Clements C, Jones S, Morriss R, Peters S, Cooper J, While D, et al. Self-harm in bipolar disorder: Findings from a prospective clinical database. J Affect Disord. 2015 Mar;173:113-9.

52. Nixon MK, Cloutier P, Jansson SM. Nonsuicidal self-harm in youth: A population-based survey. CMAJ. 2008 Jan;178(3):306-12.

53. Lenkiewicz K, Racicka E, Brynska A. Self-injury placement in mental disorders classifications, risk factors and primary mechanisms: Review of the literature. Psychiatr Pol. 2017 Apr;51(2):323-34.

54. Dunner DL, Patrick V, Fieve RR. Rapid cycling manic depressive patients. Compr Psychiatry. 1977 Nov;18(6):561-6.

55. Kukopulos A, Caliari B, Tundo A, Minnai G, Floris G, Reginaldi D, et al. Rapid cyclers, temperament, and antidepressants. Compr Psychiatry. 1983 May;24(3):249-58.

56. Coryell W, Endicott J, Keller M. Rapidly cycling affective disorder: Demographics, diagnosis, family history, and course. Arch Gen Psychiatry. 1992 Feb;49(2):126-31.

57. Baldessarini RJ, Tondo L, Floris G, Hennen J. Effects of rapid cycling on response to lithium maintenance treatment in 360 bipolar I and II disorder patients. J Affect Disord. 2000 Dec;61(1):13-22.

58. Hajek T, Hahn M, Slaney C, Garnham J, Green J, Rflzickova M, et al. Rapid cycling bipolar disorders in primary and tertiary care treated patients. Bipolar Disord. 2008 Jun;10(4):495-502.

59. Baek JH, Park DY, Choi J, Kim JS, Choi JS, Ha K, et al. Differences between bipolar I and bipolar II disorders in clinical features, comorbidity, and family history. J Affect Disord. 2011 Jun;131(1):59-67.

60. Altamura AC, Buoli M, Cesana B, Dell'Osso B, Tacchini G, Albert U, et al. Sociodemographic and clinical characterization of patients with Bipolar Disorder I vs. II: A nationwide Italian study. Eur Arch Psychiatry Clin Neurosci. 2018 Mar;268(2):169-77.

61. Coryell W, Solomon D, Turvey C, Keller M, Leon AC, Endicott J, et al. The long-term course of rapid-cycling bipolar disorder. Arch Gen Psychiatry. 2003 Sep;60(9):914-20.

62. Schneck CD, Miklowitz DJ, Miyahara S, Araga M, Wisniewski S, Gyulai L, et al. The prospective course of rapid-cycling bipolar disorder: Findings from the STEP-BD. Am J Psychiatry. 2008 Mar;165(3):370-7.

63. Chebli S. Profil evolutif du trouble bipolaire. [thesis: medicine]. Tunis: Faculte de medecine de Tunis; 2016.

64. Ben Cheikh A. Impact de la polarite du premier épisode sur revolution et le pronostic des troubles bipolaires type I et II. [thesis: medicine]. Tunis: Faculte de medecine de Tunis; 2013.

65. Cate Carter TD, Mundo E, Parikh SV, Kennedy JL. Early age at onset as a risk factor for poor outcome of bipolar disorder. J Psychiatr Res. 2003 Jul;37(4):297-303.

66. Coryell W. Rapid cycling bipolar disorder: Clinical characteristics and treatment options. CNS Drugs. 2005 Aug;19(7):557-69.

67. Ernst CL, Goldberg JF. Clinical features related to age at onset in bipolar disorder. J Affect Disord. 2004 Oct;82(1):21-7.

68. Post RM. Kindling and sensitization as models for affective episode recurrence, cyclicity, and tolerance phenomena. Neurosci Biobehav Rev. 2007 Jan;31(6):858-73.

69. Bauer MS, Calabrese JR, Dunner DL, Post R, Whybrow PC, Gyulai L, et al. Multisite data reanalysis of the validity of rapid cycling as a course modifier for bipolar disorder in DSM-IV. Am J Psychiatry. 1994 Apr;151(4):506-15.

70. Serretti A, Mandelli L, Lattuada E, Smeraldi E. Rapid cycling mood disorder: Clinical and demographic features. Compr Psychiatry. 2002 Sep;43(5):336-43.

71. Azorin JM, Kaladjian A, Adida M, Fakra E, Hantouche E, Lancrenon S. Correlates of first-episode polarity in a French cohort of 1089 bipolar I disorder patients: Role of temperaments and triggering events. J Affect Disord. 2011 Mar;129(1):39-46.

72. Perugi G, Micheli C, Akiskal HS, Madaro D, Socci C, Quilici C, et al. Polarity of the first episode, clinical characteristics, and course of manic depressive illness: A systematic retrospective investigation of 320 bipolar I patients. Compr Psychiatry. 2000 Jan;41(1):13-8.

73. Kupka RW, Luckenbaugh DA, Post RM, Nolen WA. Rapid and non-rapid cycling bipolar disorder: A meta-analysis of clinical studies. J Clin Psychiatry. 2003 Dec;64(12):1483-94.

74. Bram N, Elloumi H, Zalila H, Cheour M, Boussetta A. Clinical and evolutionary characteristics of bipolar disorder according to the polarity of the first episode. Tunis Med. 2012 May;90(5):380-6.

75. Dakhlaoui O, Essafi I, Haffani F. Clinical features of bipolar disorder: Unipolar mania: A study of patients in Tunisia. Encephale. Sept 2008;34(4):337-42.

76. Goldberg JF, Wankmuller MM, Sutherland KH. Depression with versus without manic features in rapid-cycling bipolar disorder. J Nerv Ment Dis. 2004 Sep;192(9):602-6.

77. Haro JM, VanOs J, Vieta E, Reed C, Lorenzo M, Goetz I, et al. Evidence for three distinct classes of typical, psychotic and dual mania: Results from the EMBLEM study. Acta Psychiatr Scand. 2006 Feb;113(2):112-20.

78. Gao K, Verduin ML, Kemp DE, Tolliver BK, Ganocy SJ, Elhaj O, et al. Clinical correlates of patients with rapid-cycling bipolar disorder and a recent history of substance use disorder: A subtype comparison from baseline data of 2 randomized, placebo- controlled trials. J Clin Psychiatry. 2008 Jul;69(7):1057-63.

79. Skodol AE, Grilo CM, Keyes KM, Geier T, Grant BF, Hasin DS. Relationship of personality disorders to the course of major depressive disorder in a nationally representative sample. Am J Psychiatry. 2011 Mar;168(3):257-64.

80. Friborg O, Martinsen EW, Martinussen M, Kaiser S, Overg3rd KT, Rosenvinge JH. Comorbidity of personality disorders in mood disorders: A meta-analytic review of 122 studies from 1988 to 2010. J Affect Disord. 2014 Jan;152:1-11.

81. Arici C, Cremaschi L, Dobrea C, Vismara M, Grancini B, Benatti B, et al. Differentiating multiple vs. single lifetime suicide attempters with bipolar disorders: A retrospective study. Compr Psychiatry. 2018 Jan;80:214-22.

82. Garcia-Amador M, Colom F, Valenti M, Horga G, Vieta E. Suicide risk in rapid cycling bipolar patients. J Affect Disord. 2009 Sep;117(1):74-8.

83. Bobo WV, Na PJ, Geske JR, McElroy SL, Frye MA, Biernacka JM. The relative influence of individual risk factors for attempted suicide in patients with bipolar I versus bipolar II disorder. J Affect Disord. 2018 Jan;225:489-94.

84. Undurraga J, Baldessarini RJ, Valenti M, Pacchiarotti I, Vieta E. Suicidal risk factors in bipolar I and II disorder patients. J Clin Psychiatry. 2011 Dec;72(6):778-82.

85. Gama CS, Kunz M, Magalhaes PVS, Kapczinski F. Staging and neuroprogression in bipolar disorder: A systematic review of the literature. Braz J Psychiatry. 2013 Mar;35:70-4.

86. Berk M. Neuroprogression: Pathways to progressive brain changes in bipolar disorder. Int J Neuropsychopharmacol. 2009 May;12(4):441-5.

87. Gitlin MJ. Antidepressants in bipolar depression: An enduring controversy. Int J Bipolar Disord. 2018 Dec;6(1):1-7.

88. Tondo L, Hennen J, Baldessarini RJ. Rapid-cycling bipolar disorder: Effects of long-term treatments. Acta Psychiatr Scand. 2003 Jul;108(1):4-14.

89. Calabrese JR, Shelton MD, Rapport DJ, Youngstrom EA, Jackson K, Bilali S, et al. A 20month, double-blind, maintenance trial of lithium versus divalproex in rapid-cycling bipolar disorder. Am J Psychiatry. 2005 Nov;162(11):2152-61.

90. Fountoulakis KN, Kontis D, Gonda X, Yatham LN. A systematic review of the evidence on the treatment of rapid cycling bipolar disorder. Bipolar Disord. 2013 Mar;15(2):115-37.

91. Suppes T, Brown E, Schuh LM, Baker RW, Tohen M. Rapid versus non-rapid cycling as a predictor of response to olanzapine and divalproex sodium for bipolar mania and maintenance of remission: Post hoc analyses of 47-week data. J Affect Disord. 2005 Dec;89(1):69-77.

92. Kessing LV, Andersen PK. Evidence for clinical progression of unipolar and bipolar disorders. Acta Psychiatr Scand. 2017 Jan;135(1):51-64.

93. Geller B, Craney JL, Bolhofner K, Nickelsburg MJ, Williams M, Zimerman B. Two-year prospective follow-up of children with a prepubertal and early adolescent bipolar disorder phenotype. Am J Psychiatry. 2002 Jun;159(6):927-33.

94. Gay C, Poirier MF, Olie JP. Clinical and etiopathogenetic aspects of rapid-cycle manic- depressive psychosis. Ann Med Psychol. 1987 Jan;145(1):83-90.

95. Baillarger J. Pathologie de la folie a double forme. Ann Med Psychol. July 1880;38:5-36.

96. Ritti A. Traite clinique de la folie a double forme: folie circulaire, delire a formes alternes. Paris: Doin; 1883.

97. Kraepelin E. La folie maniaque-depressive. Grenoble: Editions Jerome Millon; 1993.

98. Dunner DL. Rapid cycling bipolar manic depressive illness. Psychiatr Clin North Am. 1979 Dec;2(3):461-7.

99. Kramlinger KG, Post RM. Ultra-rapid and ultradian cycling in bipolar affective illness. Br J Psychiatry. 1996 Mar;168(3):314-23.

100. Maj M, Pirozzi R, Formicola AMR, Tortorella A. Reliability and Validity of four alternative definitions of rapid-cycling bipolar disorder. Am J Psychiatry. 1999 Sep;156(9):1421-4.

101. Bauer M, Beaulieu S, Dunner DL, Lafer B, Kupka R. Rapid cycling bipolar disorder - diagnostic concepts. Bipolar Disord. 2008 Feb;10:153-62.

102. Howland RH, Thase ME. A comprehensive review of cyclothymic disorder. J Nerv Ment Dis. 1993 Aug;181(8):485-93.

103. El-Mallakh RS, Vohringer PA, Ostacher MM, Baldassano CF, Holtzman NS, Whitham EA, et al. Antidepressants worsen rapid-cycling course in bipolar depression: A STEP-BD randomized clinical trial. J Affect Disord. 2015 Sep;184:318-21.

104. Yatham LN, Kennedy SH, Parikh SV, Schaffer A, Bond DJ, Frey BN, et al. Canadian Network for Mood and Anxiety Treatments (CANMAT) and International Society for Bipolar Disorders (ISBD) 2018 guidelines for the management of patients with bipolar disorder. Bipolar Disord. 2018 Mar;20(2):97-170.

VII.APPENDICES

Appendix 1:

Socio-demographic data

Service	□	A	
	□	B	
Dossier n : ___________	□	G	

Age :

Gender	□	Men	□	Woman
Address	□	Greater Tunis		□ Beja
	□	Bizerte		□ Seliana
	□	Rural		□ Urban
Living parents	□	Father	□	Mere
Divorced parents	□	Yes	□	No
Consanguinity of parents	□	Yes	□	No
Level of education	□	Primary		
	□	Secondary		
	□	Superior		
Professional Training	□	Yes	□	No
Professional activity	□	Yes	□	No
Income level	□	Modest		
	□	Medium		
	□	Aise		
Marital status	□	Marie		□ Single
	□	Divorce		□ Widower

Antecedents

Family background

History of disorder	□ mood	□ anxious
psychiatric	□ psychotic	□ substance use
History of suicide attempts □ Yes		□ No
Judicial record	□ Yes	□ No

Personal History

Somatic antecedents □	Epilepsy	□ Obesite
□	Demence	□ OSA
□	Diabetes	□ Dysthyroidism
□	HTA	□ Traumatic brain injury
□	Coronary artery disease	□ Other:
Substance use □	Alcohol	□ Volatile solvents
□	Cannabis	□ Amphetamines
□	Psychotropic drugs	□ No
□	Injectable substances	
History of sexual abuse □	Yes	□ No
History of abuse □	Yes	□ No
Tattoos / Self-mutilation □	Yes	□ No

Clinical data

Main diagnosis	□ TB1	□ TB2
Fast Cycles	□ With	□ No

Age at I'episode index :

Polarity of the index episode	□ Depressive	□ Manic

Number of episodes
- Maniacs :
- Hypomania :
____
- Depressives :
- Total :

Dominant polarity   □ Manic □ Depressive

Number of hospitalisations :
Average length of stay :
      Number of episodes with - With psychotic features:
                                    - With anxious distress:

-   With mixed characteristics :
-   With melancholic characteristics:
-   With atypical characteristics:
-   With catatonia :
-   Starting during the peri partum:
-   Seasonal :

Suicide attempts   □   No □   Yes (number : .)

Therapeutic data

Treatment received

□ Fluoxetine	□ Risperidone
□ Paroxetine	□ Amisulpride
□ Sertraline	□ Sulpiride
□ Escitalopram	□ Clozapine
□ Venlafaxine	□ Apriprazole
□ Amitriptyline	□ Diazepam
□ Clomipramine	□ Clonazepam
□ Anafranil	□ Lorazepam
□ Valproate	□ Bromazepam
□ Carbamazepine	□ Prazepam
□ Lamortigine	□ Alprazolam
□ Lithium	□ Pregabalin
□ Haloperidol	□ Hydroxyzine
□ Chlorpromazine	□ Promethazine
□ Levomepromazine	□ Zolpidem
□ Fluphenazine	□ ECT / RTMS
□ Olanzapine	□ Other : ___________

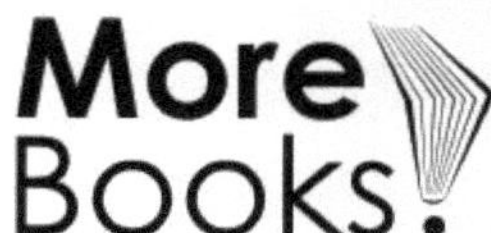

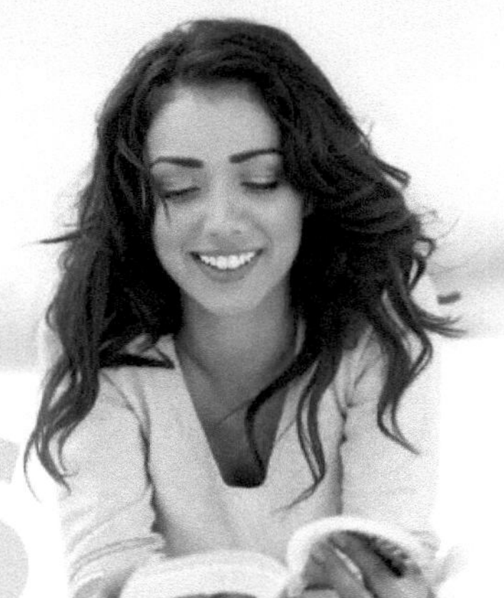

I want morebooks!

Buy your books fast and straightforward online - at one of world's fastest growing online book stores! Environmentally sound due to Print-on-Demand technologies.

Buy your books online at
www.morebooks.shop

Kaufen Sie Ihre Bücher schnell und unkompliziert online – auf einer der am schnellsten wachsenden Buchhandelsplattformen weltweit! Dank Print-On-Demand umwelt- und ressourcenschonend produziert.

Bücher schneller online kaufen
www.morebooks.shop

info@omniscriptum.com
www.omniscriptum.com

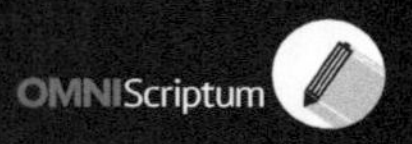
OMNIScriptum

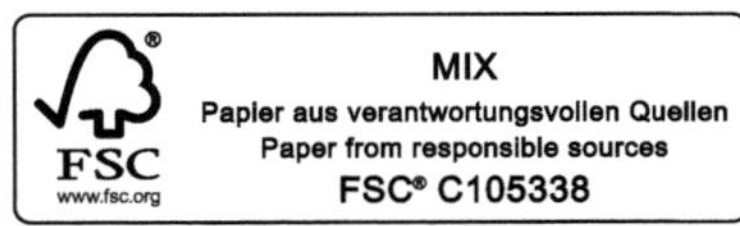

Printed by Books on Demand GmbH, Norderstedt / Germany